P9-AOU-553

Really now, why CAN'T our Johnnies READ?

JON EISENSON

PACIFIC BOOKS, PUBLISHERS
Palo Alto, California

Library of Congress Cataloging-in-Publication Data

Eisenson, Jon, 1907-
    Really now, why can't our Johnnies read? / Jon Eisenson.
       p.   cm.
    Bibliography: p.
    Includes index.
    ISBN 0-87015-258-0
    1. Literacy – United States.   2. Functional literacy – United
States.   3. Reading disability.   4. Dyslexia – United States.
I. Title.
LC151.E57 1988
372.4'145 – dc 19   88-23354
                                                                    CIP

PACIFIC BOOKS, PUBLISHERS
P.O. Box 558, Palo Alto, CA 94302-0558, U.S.A.

Preface

Why do so many of our Johnnies and a lesser number of our Joannies have so much difficulty in learning to read? Is the prevalence of reading difficulty, in degrees that range from slow, laborious, and improficient reading to virtual nonreading, as high as 20 percent, about 27 million, in our school-age and adult population? Is functional illiteracy, that is, reading no better than on a third- or fourth-grade level, as high as 13 percent in the adolescent and adult population? Are we really "A Nation at Crisis" and so "A Nation at Risk," as two recent U. S. government publications warn us? If these estimates are correct, or at least close to the mark, are they new, the result of new forces and influences? Are these estimates and their implications the consequences of recent changes in immigration to the United States? Or in our methods of teaching reading? Are there new or special influences that affect the immediate need to have proficient readers?

These are questions that I will undertake to answer in this book. But at the moment, although I do share concern with those authorities—but much less with pseudo authorities—who publicize their alarm and apprehensions, I am neither alarmed nor weighed down by anxiety about the potential of our school-age children for becoming at least as proficient in reading as their parents or teachers. I am also optimistic that the United States is not in a state of acute crisis, at least no more nor less so than other Western nations. To the degree that we may be at risk, we can and will do whatever needs to be done to minimize the hazards.

Now, let us get down to cases. "Of reading there is no end." Not quite, for unless we realize the need to teach some of our Johnnies properly—in ways they are capable of learning—the end of reading may come almost immediately after the beginning. Our Joannies are not altogether exempt from this need, but fewer of them, about one to every four of our Johnnies, are likely to fail. The unhappy consequences of inappropriate teaching we would all like to avoid. Fortunately, they can be avoided.

In this book I will identify the children who are at high risk for failure to learn to read and explain why many more Johnnies than Joannies are at risk. Alternatives to the "usual" and currently "popular" approaches to the teaching of reading will be presented that can sharply reduce the number of children who are, but need not be, denied the pleasure of learning to read and of reading for pleasure. On the negative side, I will identify the children for whom Gutenberg's invention of movable type, about 500 years earlier than the tape recorder, is an unfortunate accident of time. There is, unhappily, a very small percentage of children for whom the reading of flat print is an arduous task. This is likely to be so for any flat visual display of symbols that requires analysis for decoding for comprehension. But even these children, our "hard core" dyslexics, can learn to read well enough to meet basic intellectual needs and to become educated at the level required to join the vocations or professions of their choice. Assuming intellectual capacity, only a very few may have to settle for lesser aspirations.

JON EISENSON

Contents

Really now, why <u>CAN'T</u> our Johnnies READ?

CHAPTER ONE

What Is Reading? Basic Definitions and Statements of Personal Positions

> People are the common denominator of progress. So . . . no improvement is possible with unimproved people, and advance is certain when people are liberated and educated. . . . But we are coming to realize . . . that there is a certain sterility in economic monuments that stand alone in a sea of illiteracy. Conquest of illiteracy comes first.
>
> John Kenneth Galbraith, *Economic Development* (1964)

What may we mean by reading? Reading is making sense out of print. But this meaning is probably too restricted. For persons who have a written language that is represented by an alphabetic system, reading is decoding and deriving meaning (making sense) of printed words in context. But this is a narrow use of the word reading. Other definitions of reading include how a person may interpret and present his or her reading of a part in a play, or of a poem, or even of an abstract piece of writing. A critic who reviews the performance of an actor ("reader") may either agree or disagree with the "reading." We also have "the well-read man" or "the well-read woman" who, presumbably because of his or her wide reading, is considered a respected, knowledgeable, and sophisticated person. In a broad sense, *a reading* may be a person's interpretation of any event that is a response to the question, "What is your reading of . . . ?" And what is *your* reading of "I read you loud and clear"?

However, for the purposes of this book, the use of the term *reading* will be restricted to the *process of making sense (decoding) written material in context*. I emphasize *in context* because most single words have more than one potential meaning, and the most likely meaning becomes evident only in context. (The reader may test this observation by listing some possible meanings for the words *run, fire, red, fast, light.* Or, at random, select ten words from an unabridged dictionary.) What may be involved in the process of making sense will be considered later. For the present, note that use of the term *printed words* is avoided because many Asian-Americans employ ideographic representations (ideograms) to present ideas or events rather than an alphabetic system.

Blind persons may learn to read Braille embossings—raised dots or points—that in specified combinations stand for letters of an alphabet. These are read by finger contact. Some blind persons read puffs of air; others read vibrations. Many blind persons do much of their "reading" through listening to taped recordings.

Whatever the system, the method, or the material used for representing thought or for describing events, the common denominator meaning of *reading* is the comprehension and individual interpretation of a recorded display. The most frequent type of display is flat print. In Western cultures, the language content or message is organized into alphabetic systems of letters that constitute words. In turn, words are presented—organized—according to rules or grammars that govern their use in context.

To *decode* means to translate (transcode) from one language to another that is presumed to be the original language form in order to arrive at its meaning. When we decode, we engage in a process that has meaning as its goal. This is so whether we are transcoding from spokem to written language, or vice versa, or whether we are dealing with intentionally secret codes, or engaged in mathematical problem solving when X = a number or still another symbol, such as Y, which may have a quantitative significance. It is also so when we are involved in learning the sounds of another alphabet, such as the Greek or the augmented Greek of Russian and other Slavic languages by comparing the letters and their usual sounds with their most likely counterparts of the English alphabet.

Transcoding requires that we change the events—sights, sounds, embossings, vibrations, or whatever— from one form to another. Usually, transcoding is a step or stage toward the decoding of a message. Thus, when we sound out what a presentation of letters may suggest, we are transcoding from the visual to the articulatory-auditory, from what we see to "saying" something to ourselves that we "hear" in order to decode a message within a given context. The process of doing this with an alphabetic representation I call *phoneticizing*.

Phoneticizing means the act of producing sounds that are considered appropriate for a presentation of letters, in isolation—as single sounds, combinations of sounds, syllables, words, or in phrase or sentence context. In some languages such as Spanish, Italian, and Russian, there is a high and reliable correspondence between letters and sounds, In English, whether it is British or American English or its numerous dialects, the correspondence is neither consistent nor reliable. This should be no surprise when we recall that English has 26 letters to represent 40 to 45 sounds—vowels, consonants, and diphthongs. In any event, even though a person may be able to phoneticize (transcode from sight to sound) acceptably, unless the phoneticizer knows the meaning of what was transcoded, reading for meaning is not achieved. I have no problem in transcoding Italian and Spanish words, but I have considerable difficulty, unless a dictionary is at hand, in decoding either of these languages. The vagaries of the English language and the difficulties this language may present for easy phoneticizing wll be considered later.

Linguistic symbols are arbitrary arrangements of sounds (letters in Western language writing) that have agreed-upon meanings. Just when or how the meaning or meanings of linguistic symbols become established is often lost in history. We do know that manufacturers and their advertisers are often involved in creating new linguistic symbols— neologisms—so that listeners and viewers will associate the new words with their products.

Adolescents are among the most creative producers of new words and word combinations that, at least for a time, have common meanings to their users. *Valley speech,* a product of the late 1970s and early 1980s, is probably a combination of established slang and the hippie lingo of the 1960s. In valley speech, *bad,* properly enunciated, came to mean *good; geek* and *goober* meant weird; *rad* implied *excellent.* I give no guarantee that any of these invented or perverted words have such meanings today.

A possible exception to the arbitrariness of linguistic symbols is onomatopoetic constructions. Words such as *boom, thud, crackle, swish, ping, hiss, pop,* and *bang* presumbably suggest their meaning through the sounds we produce when we articulate them. However, linguistic symbols are not restricted to words that are produced through letter sounds. Ideograms are symbolic representations used in Chinese, Japanese, and other Oriental-Asian languages. I conjecture that if the same percentage of literacy obtained for cultures using these languages as for the cultures employing an alphabetic system, ideographic writing would be the most prevalent form throughout the world.

Reading, as noted earlier, usually involves a process of transcoding symbolic representations into another, more basic language system.

Ideographic written languages, such as Chinese, Thai, and to a considerable extent, Japanese, represent an idea or an object (at least historically) more directly than do languages that employ a written alphabetic system. Ideographic writing evokes meanings on the level of a word or phrase rather than, if transcoded, into sounds and sound sequences. Historically, ideograms may have included enough detail to be directly representational. Contemporary ideographic systems are becoming increasingly abstract and their composition—arrangement of strokes —almost as arbitrary as an arrangement of alphabetic letters into words as symbols. Thus, whether one is reading a language with an alphabetic system, or ideographs, meaning is derived by association and recalled experiences. We will consider this matter again in our brief review of written representational systems. Before this review, a few more working definitions will be offered that are relevant to this book and to my position on reading.

Reading improficiency implies a lower level of decoding (comprehension) than may be reasonably expected when such factors as opportunity, education, and other evidence of intellectual ability are considered. For example, if a 9- or 10-year-old child comprehends written language no better than a 6- or 7-year-old (assuming that he or she has been exposed to at least conventional reading instruction), the child may be considered an improficient reader. A child of secondary school age in a secondary grade who reads no better than an average third- or fourth-grade child, is certainly improficient in reading. An adolescent or adult who by most indications is of at least average intelligence and can comprehend what he or she is reading no better than a sixth-grade child is also improficient in reading. The causes of such improficiencies will be considered later. Insofar as such improficiency—semi-literacy because of the difficulties in writing usually associated with it—is accepted either by the individual or by society, we may indeed be a nation at risk.

Literacy implies the ability to read and to write (spell correctly, use acceptable grammar) on at least an average level of competence. For the present, let us consider this to be the ninth-grade level of educational achievement. In the narrowest sense, a literate person is one who can read and write at least as well as an average ninth-grade student who has earned his or her promotions to that grade. However, the term *literate* has other implications. We identify a person as literate because he or she shows evidence of a good education. Literate is also the term we use for a person who has a superior knowledge of literature and also for a person who demonstrates excellence in verbal skills, who is verbally facile, "polished," and who may be both lucid and precise in spoken or written communications.

In contrast, an illiterate person is extremely limited in these abilities, especially in reading and writing. However, there certainly are some verbally facile persons who are, at best, semi-literate.

The term *dyslexia* has too many meanings, which deprives us of significant meaning. Some "authorities" on reading equate the term with what I have explained as reading improficiency. To be sure, all dyslexics have or had difficulty in learning to read, and some continue to have difficulty as adults, but all persons who are improficient readers are not per se dyslexic. In 1969, the Interdisciplinary Committee on Reading Problems considered dyslexia to be "A disorder of children, who despite conventional classroom experience fail to attain the language skills of reading, writing, and spelling commensurate with their intellectual abilities." The Random House Dictionary defines dyslexia as "An impairment in the ability to read due to a brain deficit."

I shall define dyslexia as a severe disability of children to learn to read that is not accounted for by emotional factors, or intellectual limitation, or lack of opportunity for instruction. Dyslexic children almost always follow a familial pattern that includes learning disabilities. Dyslexia occurs three to four times as often in boys as in girls and is almost surely genetic in origin.

With these definitions and some admittedly subjective explanations out of the way (but we will return to them), some very brief historic notes on writing and its relationship to spoken language are presented below.

We do not know how speech—spoken langage—began. It can be said with a fair degree of confidence that human beings were able to use a spoken language system tens of thousands, perhaps hundreds of thousands of years, before they evolved written language. To set a very approximate date for writing, let us assume that it was no earlier than 6,000 B.C. About this time in history, writing was pictographic and so, we may assume, directly representational as to meaning. We may also assume that nonreaders either had serious visual defects or were seriously mentally retarded. Because such persons may not have had a good survival rate, we may also assume that there were no improficient readers who had an opportunity to learn to read.

Written language took either of two main courses: It either developed independently of the spoken language system, as in pictographic writing and ideographic presentations, or it developed a system that followed and corresponded to the spoken language. Either course or route had the task of symbolizing objects, events, and ideas so that the products could be taught and understood. Both systems share the need for common acceptance by their users as to the symbolic nature of the units of writing and the emergence of meanings that take place when writing—words or ideograms—is incorporated into contexts.

Japanese has taken both routes. Japanese writing combines the use of Chinese ideograms with syllabaries, which are syllables that are equivalent to the word endings in English writing that indicate grammatical features such as tense and inflectional endings on nouns, adjectives, and pronouns (see Figure 1-1).

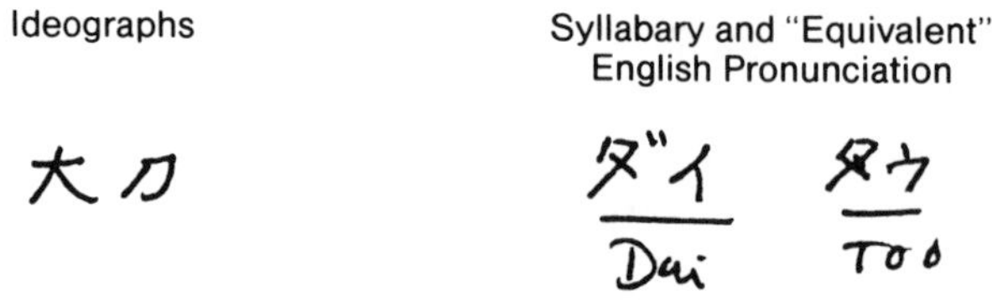

Ideographs	Syllabary and "Equivalent" English Pronunciation
大刀	ダイ タゥ
	Dai Too

FIGURE 1–1. Japanese ideograph and syllabary for "large knife."

Alphabetic languages present problems in spelling because living languages undergo changes in pronunciation that may not be consistent with the letters of the alphabet that represent them. An established national authority can dictate acceptable pronunciations or acceptable changes in spelling or grammar, as the Greeks did in 1976 and 1982. Spanish, Italian, and Russian, as already indicated, have a high consistency between spelling and pronunciation. English and French do not. Both of these languages have "frozen" the spellings of words so that, despite pronunciation changes, there is an ever-increasing distance between writing and orthographic (spelling) representation. In effect, English spelling today often tells us more about the history of a word than it guides us to its contemporary pronunciation. Examples are words such as *enough, anxious, eye, exact,* and *through.* The spellings of these words are more representative of Middle English than of contemporary letter-to-sound correspondence.

Although one can do no more than speculate when "In the beginning was the Word" can be dated, we have considerable evidence of writing in pre- and post-biblical periods. Figure 1-2 is an example of ancient pictographs and ideographic writings over a period of 3,700 years. Figure 1-3 indicates changes in ideograms intoduced by the People's Republic of China in 1956. Simplification of the characters is achieved by requiring fewer strokes for the writing of the ideograms.

Figure 1-4 shows some visual writings that are more directly representative than the Chinese ideograms. These are pictographs and

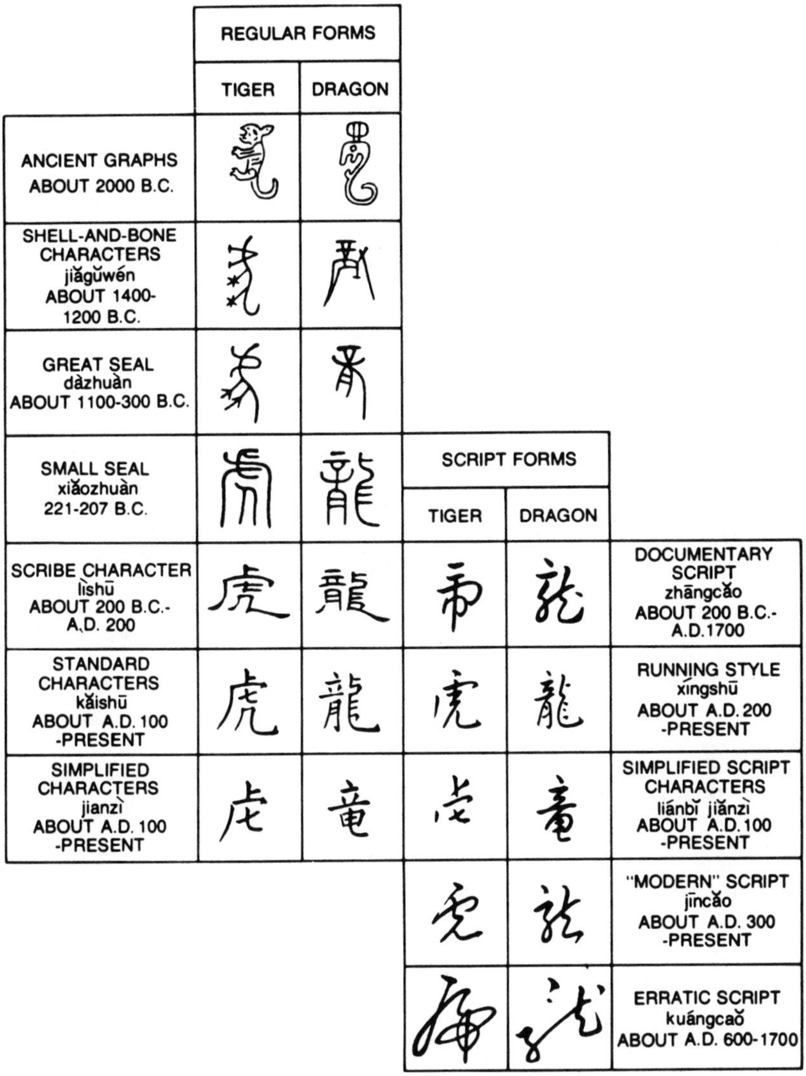

	REGULAR FORMS		SCRIPT FORMS		
	TIGER	DRAGON	TIGER	DRAGON	
ANCIENT GRAPHS ABOUT 2000 B.C.	🐅	🐉			
SHELL-AND-BONE CHARACTERS jiǎgǔwén ABOUT 1400-1200 B.C.					
GREAT SEAL dàzhuàn ABOUT 1100-300 B.C.					
SMALL SEAL xiǎozhuàn 221-207 B.C.					
SCRIBE CHARACTER lìshū ABOUT 200 B.C.-A.D. 200	虎	龍	帝	龙	DOCUMENTARY SCRIPT zhāngcǎo ABOUT 200 B.C.-A.D.1700
STANDARD CHARACTERS kǎishū ABOUT A.D.100 -PRESENT	虎	龍	虎	龍	RUNNING STYLE xíngshū ABOUT A.D.200 -PRESENT
SIMPLIFIED CHARACTERS jiǎnzì ABOUT A.D.100 -PRESENT	虍	竜	虎	童	SIMPLIFIED SCRIPT CHARACTERS liánbǐ jiǎnzì ABOUT A.D.100 -PRESENT
			虎	龙	"MODERN" SCRIPT jīncǎo ABOUT A.D. 300 -PRESENT
			屈	龙	ERRATIC SCRIPT kuángcǎo ABOUT A.D. 600-1700

FIGURE 1–2. This figure, from *Introduction to Chinese Cursive Script* by F. Y. Wang of Seton Hall University, shows some of the changes in the writing of Chinese ideograms from about 2000 B.C. to 1700 A.D. From William S-Y. Wang, "The Chinese Language," in *Human Communication*, 1982, San Francisco: W. H. Freeman and Company. Reprinted by permission.

	OLD	SIMPLIFIED
SUN (rì)	日	日
STAR (xīng)	星	星
MORNING SUN (lóng)	曨	昽
HORSE (mǎ)	馬	马
MOTHER (mā)	媽	妈
AGATE (mǎ)	瑪	玛
ANT (mǎ)	螞	蚂
TO SCOLD (mà)	罵	骂

FIGURE 1–3. Illustration of the changes in the writing of Chinese characters (ideograms) authorized by the government of the People's Republic of China in 1956. The first two characters were not changed; the others were reduced by six strokes. From William S-Y. Wang, "The Chinese Language," in *Human Communication*, 1982, San Francisco: W. H. Freeman and Company. Reprinted by permission.

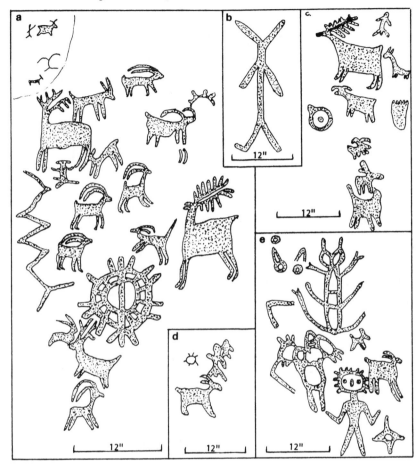

FIGURE 1–4. From *Pictographs & Petroglyphs of the Oregon Country* by T. Malcolm Loring and Louise Loring, Monograph XXI, 1982, Los Angeles: Institute of Archeology, University of California at Los Angeles. Reprinted by permission.

stone writings found in caves of Indians in the state of Washington. Figure 1-5 is a contemporary form of writing, which I had no difficulty in reading while on a vacation in Italy.

Although images for directional and "important to know" places are not internationally uniform, the number of their most likely meanings is restricted. Figure 1-6 shows how Mexico dealt with the matter of providing fairly reliable communication for visitors to the 1968 Olympic Games.

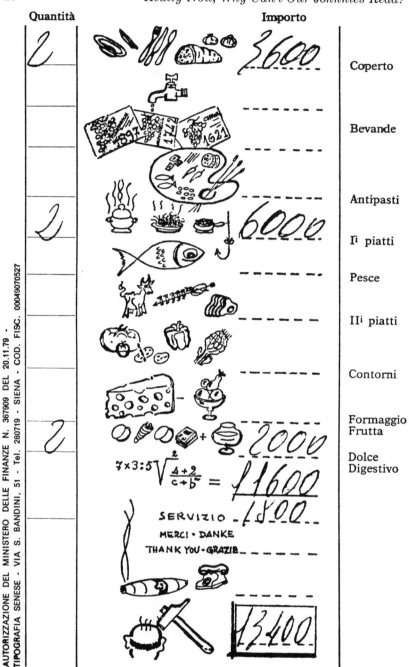

FIGURE 1–5. An Italian way of making certain that a bill is understood and paid.

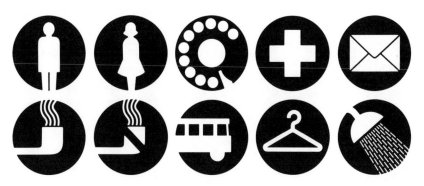

FIGURE 1–6. Some of the signs used for the 1968 Olympic Games in Mexico. Because the number of possible meanings of each sign is limited, reliable communications may be assumed. The use of signs such as these is one way of communicating to persons who cannot read an alphabetic language. E. G. Gombrich, 1972, "The Visual Image," *Scientific American*, 227, No. 3, September, 82–96. Reprinted by permission.

In a later chapter visual (nonverbal) and modified visual signs and alphabetic writing will be presented as initial or alternative approaches to the teaching of reading. I will conclude this chapter by reviewing briefly the development of alphabetic systems of writing.

Contemporary alphabets of Western Europe and of the Americas are basically Roman. Greece uses a Greek alphabet; Slavic languages employ Cyrillic (Table 1-1), an augmented Greek alphabet. Hebrew and Arabic have their own alphabets. India has many languages but for its most important writing, a system called Devanagari is used. Devanagari combines an alphabet and syllabic features.

It is likely that most contemporary alphabets can be traced to signs of Egyptian hieroglyphic writing (Figures 1-7 and 1-8). However, our concern will be the English alphabet and how well it can be used to represent the sounds of our language. For historical perspective, Figure 1-9 presents changes in Greek alphabets and "equivalents" to modern alphabets.

The International Phonetic Alphabetic symbols for the sounds of American English are included in Tables 1-2 and 1-3. The International Phonetic Alphabet (IPA) includes symbols for sounds of the principal languages of the world. Through the use of the IPA it should be possible to represent how any word may be pronounced regardless of spelling or variations of dialect. To take care of pronunciations for American English, 44 symbols are required rather than the 26 letters of the alphabet.

TABLE 1-1

EXAMPLES OF CYRILLIC WRITING (RUSSIAN)

English	Russian	Phonetic Pronunciation
1. Yes	1. Да	1. Dah
2. No	2. Нет	2. Nyet
3. Perhaps	3. Может быть	3. Mo'zhit bit'
4. Please	4. Пожапуйста	4. Pazhah'lasta
5. Thank you	5. Спасибо	5. Spasee'ba
6. Good	6. Хорошо	6. Kharasho'
7. Bad	7. Ппохо	7. Plo'kha
8. Very good	8. Очень хорошо	8. O'cheen' kharasho'
9. It is allowed	9. Можно	9. Mo'zhna
10. It is not allowed	10. Непьзя	10. Neel'zyah'
11. It is necessary	11. Нужно	11. Noo'zhna
12. It is not necessary	12. Не нужно	12. Nee noo'zhna
13. Many	13. Много	13. Mno'ga
14. Few	14. Мапо	14. Mah'la
15. Enough	15. Достаточно	15. Dastah'tachna
16. Everything	16. Все	16. Fsyo
17. Why?	17. Почему?	17. Pacheemoo'?
18. Because...	18. Потому что...	18. Patamoo' shto...
19. When?	19. Когда?	19. Kagdah'?
20. Now	20. Сейчас	20. Seechah's
21. Soon	21. Скоро	21. Sko'ra
22. Already	22. Уже	22. Oozhe'
23. Later	23. Потом	23. Pato'm
24. Where?	24. Где?	24. Gd'e?
25. There	25. Там	25. Tahm
26. Here	26. Здесь	26. Zd'es'
27. Far	27. Дапеко	27. Daleeko'
28. Near	28. бпизко	28. Blee'ska
29. Inside	29. Внутри	29. Vnootree'
30. Outside	30. Снаружи	30. Snaroo'zhi
31. Above	31. Наверху	31. Naveerkhoo'
32. Below	32. Внизу	32. Vneezoo'
33. Straight on	33. Прямо	33. Pryah'ma
34. Forward	34. Вперед	34. Fpeeryo't
35. Backward	35. Назад	35. Nazah't
36. On (to) the right	36. Направо	36. Naprah'va
37. On (to) the left	37. Напево	37. Nal'e'va
38. I do not understand	38. Я не понимаю	38. Yah nee paneemah'yoo
39. What did he say?	39. Что он сказап?	39. Shto on skazah'l?
40. Do not forget	40. Не забудь	40. Nee zaboo't'

Note: Russian has reliable letter-to-sound correspondence. Note that some letters have the same visual construction of letters of the English alphabet but have different sound values. What are the Russian sounds for the letters H, C, B, and Я? From *PSC Trip Information Manual*, 1978. Oceanside, NY: Professional Seminar Consultants. Reprinted by permission.

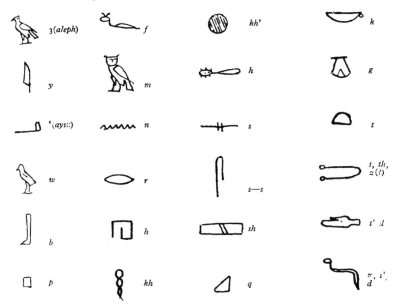

FIGURE 1–7. Earliest hieroglyphic consonantal signs ("alphabet"?). From *The Alphabet: A History of Mankind* by David Diringer, 1948, New York: Philosophical Library, Inc. Reprinted by permission.

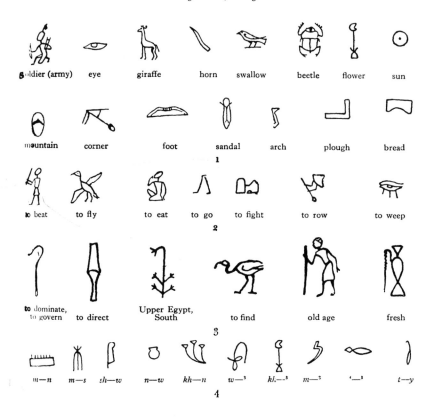

soldier (army)   eye   giraffe   horn   swallow   beetle   flower   sun

mountain   corner   foot   sandal   arch   plough   bread

1

to beat   to fly   to eat   to go   to fight   to row   to weep

2

to dominate,   to direct   Upper Egypt,   to find   old age   fresh
to govern   South

3

m—n   *m—s*   *sh—w*   *n—w*   *kh—n*   *w—ᵓ*   *kl.—ᵓ*   *m—ᵓ*   *ᶜ—ᵓ*   *t—y*

4

FIGURE 1–8. Hieroglyphic word-signs. From *The Alphabet: A History of Mankind* by David Diringer, 1948, New York: Philosophical Library, Inc. Reprinted by permission.

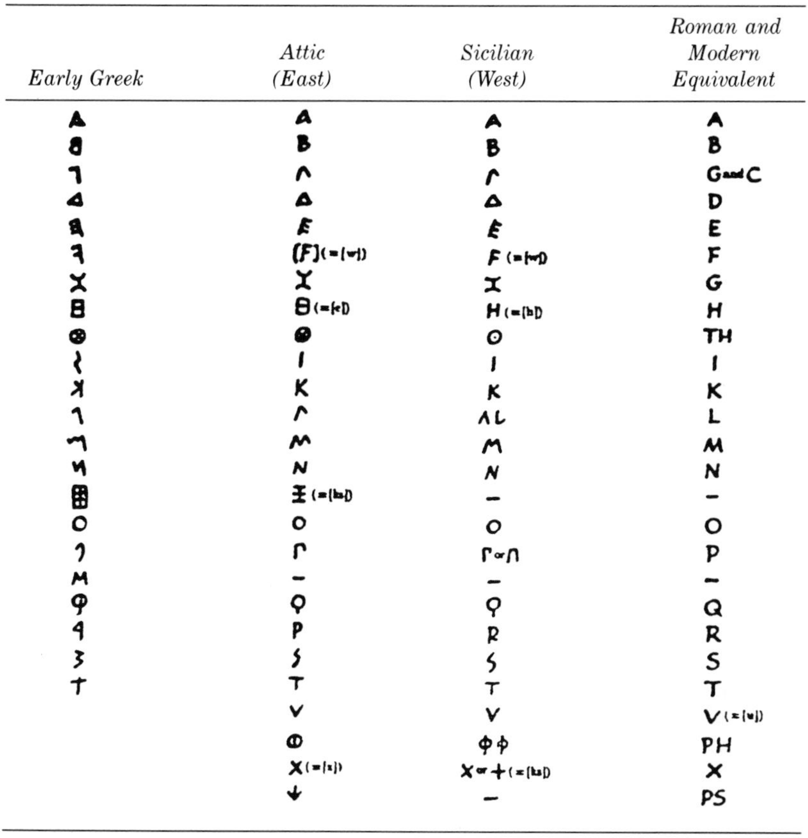

Early Greek	Attic (East)	Sicilian (West)	Roman and Modern Equivalent
A	A	A	A
B	B	B	B
ʌ	∧	ↄ	G and C
◁	△	△	D
⅃	E	E	E
⅂	(F)(=⟨v⟩)	F (=⟨w⟩)	F
X	X	X	G
B	B(=⟨h⟩)	H(=⟨h⟩)	H
⊕	⊕	O	TH
⟨	I	I	I
X	K	K	K
⅂	↗	∧L	L
⌐	M	M	M
N	N	N	N
⊞	Ξ(=⟨ks⟩)	—	—
O	O	O	O
⟩	Γ	Γ or ∩	P
M	—	—	—
φ	φ	φ	Q
9	P	R	R
ζ	ζ	ξ	S
T	T	T	T
	V	V	V (=⟨u⟩)
	Φ	φ φ	PH
	X(=⟨x⟩)	X or + (=⟨h⟩)	X
	↓	—	PS

FIGURE 1–9. Greek alphabets, early and contemporary, and some modern (mostly Roman) equivalents.

TABLE 1-2

THE COMMON PHONEMES OF AMERICAN ENGLISH (CONSONANTS)

Key Word	Most Frequent Dictionary Symbol	IPA Symbol
1. *p*at	p	p
2. *b*ee	b	b
3. *t*in	t	t
4. *d*en	d	d
5. *c*ook	k	k
6. *g*et	g	g
7. *f*ast	f	f
8. *v*an	v	v
9. *th*in	th	θ
10. *th*is	~~th~~, *th*	ð
11. *s*ea	s	s
12. *z*oo	z	z
13. *sh*e	sh	ʃ
14. trea*s*ure	zh	ʒ
15. *ch*ick	ch	tʃ
16. *j*ump	j	dʒ
17. *m*e	m	m
18. *n*o	n	n
19. si*ng*	ng	ŋ
20. *l*et	l	l
21. *r*un	r	r
22. *y*ell	y	j
23. *h*at	h	h
24. *w*on	w	w
25. *wh*at	hw	ʍ or hw

Note: From *Voice and Diction*, 5th ed. by J. Eisenson, 1983. New York: Macmillan Publishing Co.

TABLE 1-3

THE COMMON PHONEMES OF AMERICAN ENGLISH (VOWELS)

Key Word	Dictionary Symbol	IPA* Symbol
26. fee	ē	i
27. sit	ĭ	ɪ
28. take	ā	e
29. met	ĕ	ɛ
30. cat	ă	æ
31. task	ă or a·	æ or a depending upon regional or individual variations
32. calm	ä	a
33. hot	ŏ or ä	ɒ or a depending upon regional or individual variations
34. saw	ô	ɔ
35. vote	ō	o or ou
36. bull	o͝o	ʊ
37. too	o͞o	u
38. hut	ŭ	ʌ
39. about	ə	ə
40. upper	ər	ɝ by most Americans and ə by many others
41. bird	ûr	ɝ by most Americans and ɝ by many others
Phonemic Diphthongs		
42. ice	ī	aɪ
43. now	ou	aʊ or ɑʊ
44. boy	oi	ɔɪ

*International Phonetic Alphabet.

Note: From *Voice and Diction*, 5th ed. by J. Eisenson, 1983. New York: Macmillan Publishing Co.

CHAPTER TWO

Reading Failure and Functional Illiteracy in the United States

The biggest threat to the Constitution of the United States may be the 20 million Americans who can't read it.*

★ ★ ★ ★ ★

Reading maketh a full man, conference a ready man, and writing an exact man.

Francies Bacon, *Of Studies*

In the Preface it was stated that reading improficiency and reading failure—severe deficiency in reading not associated with lack of opportunity or the need to learn to read—is as high as 20 percent in the United States. Because of this, we are considered by many educators and perhaps even more by our sensitive politicians to be "A Nation at Crisis" and "A Nation at Risk." I am not as alarmed by these reports as are some of my colleagues, because there are causes for this situation that can be identified and, fortunately, corrected.

First, we need to understand that today functional illiteracy, and even the inability or virtual inability to read and to write, may still be, as it long has been, related to a lack of opportunity and possibly a lack of motivation. These causes are not as prevalent in the United States and most Western nations as they are in the Third World countries, but they still exist. We do have adults who have emigrated to the United States, legally as well as illegally, who were illiterate in their first (native) language. All too often, as agricultural and manual laborers, they find

---

*Wording of the headline of an advertisement in the *New York Times*, Sunday, August 31, 1986. The advertisement continues, "What happens to a democracy when millions of its citizens cannot read its Constitution? What price does society pay when millions of adults struggle with even basic tasks, such as filling out job applications or reading simple instructions?"

neither opportunity nor economic reward to become literate. In some instances, they do learn to read and to write and to become more completely educated despite discouraging circumstances. Children of migrant workers have interrupted educational histories that are reflected in low educational achievement. To be sure, these children do not compose a significant number of our total population, but they are not to be ignored.

Other Americans, for a variety of reasons, lack the motivation or opportunity to become literate. It is unlikely that many of these Americans are incapable of learning to read and to write. However, most children who, for whatever reason, do not learn to read and to write, do not fall into ready-made categories that account for or even identify the causes of their disability. Such school-age children, in primary, middle, and secondary grades, and some adults who are "disabled readers" are found in all levels of intelligence in all cultural and socioeconomic groups. They are members of intact families and of broken homes. Some have strict disciplinarians as parents and others have or had permissive ones. In their book *Reading Disability*, Florence Roswell and Gladys Natchez (1977) note that:

> In some instances a child with reading problems shows severe emotional difficulty at the outset; sometimes the maladjustment manifests itself only after the appearance of poor achievement. But all children with reading disability manifest some disequilibrium in their lives. (p. 5)

However much I agree with the general observations of Drs. Roswell and Natchez, there are still other children who are at high risk for failure *because they are different* in ways that we will consider later. But first we will examine the matter of functional illiteracy. Then the prevalence of such reading improficiency in the United States will be compared with that in other countries and other cultures.

FUNCTIONAL ILLITERACY: AN EXPANDED CONSIDERATION

The recent United States government publications referred to at the beginning of this chapter—"A Nation at Crisis" and "A Nation at Risk"—might give the impression that the present high rate of reading improficiency—possibly as high as 20 percent—and the rate of functional illiteracy—as high as 13 percent—are new problems. They are not. They have existed for at least one hundred years. However, this "discovery" has more serious implications today than at any time in our country's history. Our national needs no longer permit us to indulge ourselves with functional illiteracy or even a lesser degree of reading improficiency.

Functional illiteracy is a relative term that cannot be divorced from the needs and legitimate expectations of a society. Thus, functional illiteracy may be considered the minimal level of ability to read and to write that a given society considers acceptable. In the United States, a person might be considered functionally illiterate if he cannot read the intended messages in his local newspaper, or find a listed number in a telephone directory, or look up the meaning of a word in a dictionary. Unless the application form is intentionally complicated, an elementary school graduate should be able to fill out the form to apply for a position, or obtain telephone service, or open a credit account. According to other criteria, a person might be considered functionally illiterate if he or she at age 12 cannot understand what is presented in a well-written third- or fourth-grade reader. I would not, however, consider an adult functionally illiterate if he or she is not able to figure out why the IRS is imposing a penalty for alleged underpayment of taxes or even, less frequently, about to surprise the taxpayer with a refund for overpayment.

FUNCTIONAL ILLITERACY IN OTHER COUNTRIES

With due allowance for differences according to national and cultural needs and expectations, where do we stand? As indicated earlier, we have once again "discovered" that about 13 percent of our population is functionally illiterate. In Japan, this figure is reported to be a mere 1 percent. The low estimates may be related either to national pride, or to the selection of those who are included in the statistics. If, for a predetermined reason, children who are not expected to learn to read are not included in those who are taught, we will have a very different set of figures than we would have when all school-age children are included in the data. In the Scandinavian countries, it is about 5 percent. In China, it is about 25 percent. In sharp contrast, at least 95 percent of the black population of Africa, undoubtedly for lack of opportunity, is illiterate. In rural areas of Southern Europe—Spain, Portugal, and Italy—about 50 percent of the population is functionally illiterate. In the Soviet Union, I have been informed by a member of the research staff of the Moscow Institute of Defectology, 20 percent of children have difficulty in learning to read when they begin formal instruction at age 7. However, by age 10, all who are taught are able to read. Again, this observation may reflect national pride, and perhaps an unwillingness or at least a reluctance to admit possible failure. (Most of the estimates are from Young & Tyre, 1983.)

Now, understanding that in some major cultures and subcultures, a limited amount of literacy is all that is needed to meet expectations, we will consider the chief causes of reading disability in the United States. Insofar as we may assume opportunity and motivation to learn to read to be acceptable, the causes for reading disability (improficiency) are not peculiar to the United States. In the presentation that follows, possible environmental, cultural, educational factors will be considered separately from individual physical and intellectual causes, although in many instances they are associated and interrelated.

READING ENVIRONMENT

A good reading environment is a home in which family members not only have books and magazines and other reading materials, but spend some time in reading them. This setting establishes the notion that reading is a worth-while and enjoyable activity. Having reading material but ignoring it establishes the opposite attitude. A family environment in which parents, older siblings, or other relatives read to young children to share pleasure and information is definitely favorable for the child who has not yet learned to read, as well as for the child who is a beginning reader but still enjoys being read to.

Homes such as those just described are by no means restricted to the middle or upper classes or to the socioeconomically advantaged. In economic terms, some families who are by legal definition on the poverty level provide their children with the riches of books and shared attention to them. In contrast, there are culturally impoverished homes at all socioeconomic levels. A television set, even though set for "Sesame Street," is not an adequate substitute for books and adults who enjoy reading and have the reward of children who relate warmly to those who like to read to them. To generalize, though some "disadvantaged" homes may be restricted in the availability of reading material and opportunity to read, self-imposed restrictions operate in homes at all socioeconomic levels. Though not frequent, self-imposed restrictions may also operate on all educational levels, in bilingual as well as monolingual homes. Only when the home environment does not provide proper nutrition, when children as well as adults are in poor health, emotionally or physically, do we have negative factors for reading. We also have negative factors in homes in which there is lack of opportunity or desire on the part of parents to relate to children, to nurture their intellectual and social needs. In such homes we find a direct relationship between socioeconomic level and reading improficiency.

THE LANGUAGE OF THE HOME

In this discussion we are not concerned with what language a child hears in the home, or whether the home is bilingual or monolingual, but with how language is used for communication and the expression of feelings. There is no way to ensure that every child who has concerned and caring parents will be a proficient reader. However, it is possible to describe some features of homes in which there is an increased likelihood that children will be positively inclined to and "take to" reading. To begin with, children should be exposed to spoken language that provides pleasurable communication. In a broad but by no means literal sense, the language that children listen to and overhear becomes the basis of what they will reencode when they learn to read. The alternate statement is that when a child begins to read for meaning rather than for the fun of just sounding out, he or she will use his or her knowledge of language to arrive at meanings. Spoken language that is impoverished grammatically, that includes a disproportionate amount of "biologically incompatible" utterances that are spoken for emphasis or to express negative feelings will be of no help for the beginning reader.

I am not suggesting that all conversations in homes need to be carried out in "Standard" American English and in complete and "correct" grammatical constructions. It is not necessary for a child to hear in response to a question such as "Where is your book?" the statement "The book is on my desk." The incomplete but conversational form "On my desk" is sufficient. Of course, it does no harm when speaking to a child to use grammatically complete statements, but relaxed conversations should not be made to suffer at the mercy of pedantic grammar or pedantic grammarians.

In 1961, following a study, Basil Bernstein, a British sociolinguist wrote a report which, if taken literally, seemed to indict the lower socioeconomic classes for the use of inferior language, of "restricted" codes. Such language expressed emotions at the expense of communicating information and ideas. If this is the situation, or to the degree that it might be, children from such environments are ill equipped for school learning and for learning to read in particular. In contrast, Bernstein noted that upper-class children are exposed to language that is detailed, informative, and well constructed.

Although it would be unrealistic to deny that some children from lower socioeconomic classes do need more help than most children from more advantaged homes, sweeping generalizations in either direction should not be accepted. The Headstart program launched during the 1960s is a realistic response to the language and related needs of some underprivileged preschool children.

EDUCATION AND EDUCATORS

Much reading improficiency results from teaching children at the wrong time, by the wrong persons, or by inappropriate methods. When, by whom, and how to introduce reading instruction are critical matters.

It is important for parents to provide the type of environment for reading discussed earlier. However, it is *not* wise for parents to be responsible for formal instruction in reading for their own children, even when they are professional teachers who are responsible for teaching other parents' children. When a parent engages in formal teaching of his or her child, neither is likely to maintain objectivity. In some instances there may be parents who are fully capable of whatever "formal" teaching needs to be done to introduce the child to decode written language for meaning, but they are likely to be the exception rather than the rule. The risks of emotional responses, hard to conceal expressions of disappointment and of impatience, unwillingness of the child to participate, all argue against having a parent act as teacher in a formal sense. Another point to consider is that all children within the same family are not necessarily ready to be taught to read at the same age. Success with one child is no guarantee of success with another. However, these reservations do not preclude the advantages of giving children the opportunity to have parents read to them or to provide them with books to look at and enjoy or to look at while they listen to a grown-up do the reading.

THE TEACHER AND THE METHOD

The professional teacher of reading should not be limited to any one approach or method, however successful that one may be for most children, in providing formal instruction. In most instances, the first professional teacher is the classroom teacher. Although most children can learn to read with an acceptable degree of competence without much regard to the specifics of any given method, some children, perhaps as many as 20 percent and surely no fewer than 5 percent, will not and do not. These children need approaches and methods and timing (when to begin) that are related to their neuropsychological make-up and maturation, to their individual styles of learning, and to their capacities (limits) for attending when they are formally taught. It is unfortunate that many teachers are themselves victims of "in vogue" methods that are imposed on them. It is also unfortunate that some teachers insist on one selected method for all of their pupils. Such persons are obviously the wrong persons to teach reading.

We all know of children who somehow learned to read—to decode (understand) written material—as early as age 3. We also know of children who failed to learn to read—to make any sense out of written material—until 9 years of age, and others, including high school graduates, who continue to be functionally illiterate as adults. Is there any common factor that can predict either success or failure? There is no "hard" factor, but there is a "not so soft" relationship between age when formal teaching is initiated and incidence of success. In schools in which formal reading instruction is not introduced until age 7, the percentage of reading disability is as low as 4 or 5 percent rather than the 20 percent often cited for the United States. As already noted, this is the situation in the Scandinavian countries, in Finland, and in the Soviet Union. These countries are by no means at one in regard to the method used to teach reading! There is, however, a common assumption in the countries that have a comparatively low rate of reading failure that meaning must be established at the outset; otherwise, *whatever else the child may be doing while being taught is not reading.* I also believe that the age of formal instruction—age 7 or later if the child does not "take to" reading—allows for additional time for neuropsychological maturation and so for readiness for the complex processes that are involved in learning to read for meaning. These will be considered later with due awareness that we are just beginning to learn what the neuropsychology and psycholinguistics of reading may be.

At a minimum, we need to appreciate that *the printed word is not directly equivalent to the spoken word.* Nevertheless, a child must understand a spoken language before he or she can learn to read. For most of us, the spoken code is produced orally, but for the deaf it may be a visual (manually produced) system. Although there is an important relationship between spoken and written language, between speaking and reading, there is a distance, if not a gulf, that must be bridged if we expect a child to learn to read for meaning. Anything short of arriving at meaning is, of course, not true reading.

EARLY TEACHING AND SOME POSSIBLE CONSEQUENCES

Sputnik, an artificial satellite, was launched into space on October 4, 1957 by the Soviet Union. The United States launched Explorer I on

January 31, 1958. However, this success was not sufficient to assuage our apprehensions that the USSR was dangerously ahead of us in space science and possibly in other unidentified areas of science. The pressure to introduce academic subject matter in the kindergarten may well be a result of American "Post-Sputnik" anxieties. The recent warnings of federal committees that the United States is "A Nation at Crisis" have increased pressure to initiate academic teaching, and particularly reading, in the kindergarten year. In many public schools and not a few private preschools, 5-year-old children are spending much of their day with their noses in books. They are making marks in workbooks, learning to write, and making appropriate sounds in response to sights to show that they are learning phonics as part of their instruction in reading skills. Some children do, in fact, learn to read before they enter the first grade. Others do not. Among those who do not are likely to be youngsters at least as bright as those who are successful. The consequences for those who are not successful may, in some instances, be adverse and long standing.

In an article entitled "Kindergarten: Starting Older and Wiser," (*New York Times*, November 20, 1986), Sue Mittenthal reports on surveys in the New York City area of the practice of accelerated academic teaching and the effects on some of the children in both public and private schools. Some of the effects include reverting to bed-wetting, thumb sucking, and infantile speech. A few of the children had headaches that were chronic except on nonschool days. A few accepted their classmates' pronouncements that they were stupid. Others felt that they were friendless and would like to stay home and play.

Happily, this is not the situation in all schools. An increasing number of private schools are not accepting children for their kindergarten classes until they are almost 6 years of age. Mittenthal reports that ". . . a growing body of research indicates that children who are close to six years old upon entering kindergarten tend to receive better grades and score higher on achievement tests through school than those who began kindergarten having just turned five." Specifically in reference to reading, there is no evidence to suggest that children who learn to read at age 5 are any better at reading by the time they are in the third grade, at approximately age 8, than the "late starters." Whatever evidence is available makes it clear that initiating formal reading instruction at age 7 or later, as in the Scandinavian countries, results in far fewer reading failures than we acknowledge. Postponing teaching of reading until children are "older and wiser" will be considered in Chapters Five and Six.

CHAPTER THREE

Approaches and Models for Teaching Reading

You write with ease to show your breeding,
But easy writing is cursed hard reading.

Richard Brinsley Sheridan, *Clio's Protest*

How best to teach reading has been a long-standing controversy. All too often proponents and opponents of various positions generate more heat than light in their arguments. Because a majority of children seem to be able to learn to read without regard to the method by which they were supposedly taught, the arguing continues with little evidence of mutual understanding or even respect for differences in position. Recent research has provided some information on the comparative efficacy of current methods, but not enough to settle whatever the issues may be. Frankly, we still are not in agreement as to what constitutes basic skills, or the value of so-called reading readiness programs, or even when a child should be considered ready for formal instruction in reading.

Whatever the basics for reading may be, the goal of reading is undeniably the ability to comprehend a written text. I believe that basics in formal instruction should include establishing the skills and techniques and providing sufficient information about language to enable a child to decode written content for meaning(s). From my point of view, to be minimally adequate, a teaching method must provide the following:

1. Establish a vocabulary that is useful for a child to know as he or she explores the wonders of the written code.
2. Help to establish the grammatical (syntactical) structure of language.
3. Make provision for the awareness of memory in the process of identifying words and their likely meaning in a given context.

4. Allow for anticipating (predicting) what the meaning of "new" words and words "not yet read" may be in the light of the overall content.

A first approach to reading should, as early as possible, include all of the requirements above. However, it is possible to make a case for an initial approach to formal instruction in reading to omit or even discourage my fourth requirement. Certainly, the proponents of the phonic approach do not approve of guessing at words. But I strongly urge that "guessing" in the light of context is what the decoding of both spoken and written language is and what we all do or should do if we would not be forever doomed to be very slow listeners and very slow and slavish readers.

For a moderate and objective evaluation of reading approaches, with emphasis on the phonic model, see Chall (1983a). Also recommended is Williams (1979), who reviews the virtues and shortcomings of contemporary reading methods and summarizes recent research on reading. She looks forward to continuing reading instruction into the middle grades (4 to 6) to move the child beyond the teaching of "basics" in the first three grades.

In this chapter some of the current approaches to the teaching of reading will be reviewed. These approaches seem to work with about 80 percent of our primary-grade children. In this review I will explain my strong reservations about the so-called phonic approach to the teaching of reading.

The *phonic approach* assumes that if a child is taught "the sounds the letters make," it then will become possible to go directly from letters → (to) → (to) sounds → (to) sound blends that constitute the pronunciation of words → (to) meanings. However, unless the transpositions produce an inner response that evokes meaning, even if the sounding out is successful, the child has transcoded but has not decoded the arrangement of letters to deserve to be called reading.

THE PITFALLS OF ENGLISH SPELLING

Earlier I indicated that English spelling tells us more about the history of English words than how to spell them. In addition to all the historical forces that created British English, the American product also reflects Dutch, Spanish, French, and Indian influences. The results are differences in pronounciation, differences in word usage (different meanings for the same word-forms, as well as different words for the same meanings, as, for example, boot and trunk for the space in the back of an automobile; tube and subway; lorry and truck; cinema and movies). Perhaps that is in part what George Bernard Shaw implied by his observation that, "Great Britain and America are two great countries divided by the same language."

American English has an alphabet with 26 letters that somehow must represent 44 basic sounds (phonemes). These were listed earlier in Table 1-2. The basic sounds comprise 15 vowels, 5 vowel blends (diphthongs), and 24 consonants. There are rules that may inform us when letters and combinations of letters such as *c* and *s* and *g* and digraphs such as *ea* and *ue* "diverge" from their "expected" pronunciations; there are rules— considerably more than a hundred—that account for silent *k*, and *l*, and *r*, but few of us remember them when we spell the words that we need to write. We manage the pronunciation and spellings of words such as *dough, enough, through,* and *bough* through memory rather than recall of an appropriate rule. The child who learns to read proficiently sight-reads these and thousands of other words and decides on the meaning according to the context in which they occur.

To return to the pitfalls of written English and the relationship of letters to sounds, let us consider a few spellings for the sound usually represented by the letter *sh.* Spellings include *nation, precious, anxious, sugar, bush, patient, machine,* and *mission.* With a substantial knowledge of language and the ways of the world, it should be possible to transcode and decode the verses that follow for pronunciations and meaning:

> In his conscious fashion
> Cautiously Sean rationed
> His unburnished passion.

> "Pshaw," thought Lucretia,
> Who had her own notion
> Of how Sean should fashion
> His expression of devotion.

Following are some words chosen from the most frequently used in American English that illustrate differences in the pronunciation of vowel sounds. Our language has 15 vowel sounds but only *a, e, i, o, u,* and sometimes *y* to represent them. For the initial *a* we have *add, and, age, always, art,* and *ask.* For *a* in a medial position we have *back, became, day, father,* and *half* (at least three pronunciations according to regional dialect). The letter *e* provides us with *each, end, English,* and *eye.* In addition, we have the potent but silent *e* as in *life, rope, hide, pace.* But we also have *give* and *live,* the latter with two pronunciations and related meanings according to context. Thus we may write, "Live to give and thrive to be alive." The letter *o* offers *of*, *old*, *order*, *olive*, *one*, *orange* (how many pronunciations?), *originate* (contrast this with *origin*), and *ought*. I can, of course, provide examples of varying letter-to-sound correspondences for the remainder of the letters—*i*, *o*, *u*, and *y*, which is sometimes a vowel and sometimes silent. But there is no need to strain the point.

The letters to represent the consonants also have ways of their own. The letter *b* is moderately reliable except when it is silent, as in *doubt* and *debt*, *lamb* and *comb*. For the letter *c* we have *cent*, *come*, *character*, *cell*, and *cello*. This letter is also part of the digraph *ch*, as in *child*, *chain*, and *much*. But despite their spelling, the words *chaos*, *character* are not digraphs phonetically. In *chic*, *chevron*, *Cheyenne*, and *chauffeur* we have four words that reflect a French influence. The letter *l* is usually dependable, but it falls silent in *palm* and *psalm*, and has quite a different quality in *million* and *bullion*. The letter *r* is reliable in the initial position, may be silent in *harm* and *farm*, and really becomes different in both the American and British pronunciations of words such as *very*, *burn*, *yearn*, and *firm*. According to regional dialect, it may or may not be silent in *upper*, *farm*, and *danger*. There are "errant" pronunciations for many of the other letters, but the point has been made. Over all, the correspondence between letters and sounds in American English—the graphemic to phonemic correspondence—is about 50 to 60 percent for the 1,000 words most frequently used. This estimate is based on a statistical study by Eisenson and Solomon (1970). Low-frequency words tend to undergo less change and have a higher correspondence.

A child who can read—pronounce and understand—a warning, such as "Danger, thin ice, hole, no fishing allowed," probably needs to use sight-word memory and context to decode for meaning. The British writers, Young and Tyre, in their provocative book *Dyslexia or Illiteracy?* (1983) sum up their views of the relationship between print and sound by observing that:

> The complexity of the relationships between print and sound is such that the more thoroughly children master simple letter-sound associations the more they must unlearn as they proceed (p. 45).

As a general criticism of the phonic model, Young and Tyre say:

> Apart from the difficulties of going from letters to sounds to words the (phonic) model is inadequate in that it fails to account for all the work that has to be done by memory before the words can have meaning (p. 45).

Even the most ardent advocates of the phonic approach admit the need for establishing a sight vocabulary—words that can be recognized and presumably decoded for meaning in context—without sounding them out. Professor E. W. Dolch of the University of Illinois provided such a list and it is still in wide use (1960). The Dolch list includes such words as *a, about, around, big, black, far, fast, get, gave, had, has, I, if, is, its, jump, laugh, light, made, myself, never, new, not, of, off, only, pick, play, please, ran, read, said, saw, shall, take, thank, today, under, up, very, walk, want, when, where, yellow,* and *yes.* A second Dolch list includes 95 most common nouns. This list has the entries *apple, baby, cake, day, egg, farm, game, home, kitty, letter, man, name, paper, rabbit, Santa Claus, table, thing,* and *watch.*

Johnson (1971) updated the Dolch list and developed a basic sight vocabulary of 220 words that children should know on sight when they begin to learn to read (Table 3-1). About the same time, Harris and Jacobson (1972) published a list of about 5,000 words that were computer determined from a compilation of words that were used three or more times in readers in current use from the first through the sixth grade. A second Harris and Jacobson list for beginning readers—core words—includes selections of 58 preprimer, 63 primer, and 212 first-reader words.

Core words are words that children should know by sight, without need to transcode (sound out). Sight words permit a child to read with fluency and with an immediate sense of meaning.

STAGES IN READING

Chall (1983), an ardent advocate of the phonic approach as an initial stage in learning to read, proposes that there are five successive stages in learning to read and a prereading stage, from birth to age 6—the beginning of formal education in the United States. In the Prereading Stage, children acquire language and learn words and syntax. They also gain insights into the nature of words, "That some sound the same as their ends or beginnings (rhyme and alliteration), that they can be broken into parts, and that the parts can be put together (synthesized, blended) to form whole words." This stage, and the five successive formal stages, are related to children's cognitive development. Briefly stated, following are the highlights of the five successive stages:

Stage 1. Children in the first and second grades of school in the United States (ages 6–7) are taught decoding—learning the names and sounds

TABLE 3-1

BASIC WORD SIGHT VOCABULARY

Preprimer	Primer	First	Second	Third
1. the	45. when	89. many	133. know	177. don't
2. of	46. who	90. before	134. while	178. does
3. and	47. will	91. must	135. last	179. got
4. to	48. more	92. through	136. might	180. united
5. a	49. no	93. back	137. us	181. left
6. in	50. if	94. years	138. great	182. number
7. that	51. out	95. where	139. old	183. course
8. is	52. so	96. much	140. year	184. war
9. was	53. said	97. your	141. off	185. until
10. he	54. what	98. may	142. come	186. always
11. for	55. up	99. well	143. since	187. away
12. it	56. its	100. down	144. against	188. something
13. with	57. about	101. should	145. go	189. fact
14. as	58. into	102. because	146. came	190. through
15. his	59. than	103. each	147. right	191. water
16. on	60. them	104. just	148. used	192. less
17. be	61. can	105. those	149. take	193. public
18. at	62. only	106. people	150. three	194. put
19. by	63. other	107. Mr.	151. states	195. thing
20. I	64. new	108. how	152. himself	196. almost
21. this	65. some	109. too	153. few	197. hand
22. had	66. could	110. little	154. house	198. enough
23. not	67. time	111. state	155. use	199. far
24. are	68. these	112. good	156. during	200. took
25. but	69. two	113. very	157. without	201. head
26. from	70. may	114. make	158. again	202. yet
27. or	71. then	115. would	159. place	203. government
28. have	72. do	116. still	160. American	204. system
29. an	73. first	117. own	161. around	205. better
30. they	74. any	118. see	162. however	206. set
31. which	75. my	119. men	163. home	207. told
32. one	76. now	120. work	164. small	208. nothing
33. you	77. such	121. long	165. found	209. night
34. were	78. like	122. get	166. Mrs.	210. end
35. her	79. our	123. here	167. thought	211. why
36. all	80. over	124. between	168. went	212. called
37. she	81. man	125. both	169. say	213. didn't
38. there	82. me	126. life	170. part	214. eyes
39. would	83. even	127. being	171. once	215. find
40. their	84. most	128. under	172. general	216. going
41. we	85. made	129. never	173. high	217. look
42. him	86. after	130. day	174. upon	218. asked
43. been	87. also	131. same	175. school	219. later
44. has	88. did	132. another	176. every	220. knew

Note: From "The Dolch list re-examined" by D. D. Johnson, 1971, *The Reading Teacher, 24*, 455-456. Reprinted by permission.

of letters and associating them with "Corresponding parts of spoken words."

Stage 2. Usual ages, 7–8, grades 2–3. Children confirm what they know about printed words, and become "unglued from the print." If they succeed in the "ungluing," they increase in fluency of reading.

Stage 3. Ages 9–14, grades 4–8. Children read to "learn the new." Through reading they gain new knowledge, information, and vicarious experiences.

Stage 4. High school level, usual ages 14–18. Students learn to deal with a variety of viewpoints, "To deal with layers of facts and concepts added on to those acquired earlier." This is in contrast to the single point of view they are likely to be offered in textbooks in the elementary school grades. "Without the basic knowledge acquired in Stage 3, reading materials with multiple viewpoints would be difficult."

Stage 5. College-age level. Students as adults, and adults who may no longer formally be students, read selectively according to their individual purpose. Reading is constructive in that by reading what others write, the reader constructs his or her own knowledge.

For a detailed presentation of the stages of reading, see Chall (1983). Chall (1983) does not consider her reading development stages to be prescriptive. "They are meant to be rough estimates of expected progress for typical individuals—not for all individuals, nor for all times" (p. 175).

Despite her strong advocacy of the phonic approach as an initial stage in learning to read, Chall cautions that:

> If children are "Too glued to the print," without help in freeing themselves from it, they may not develop as rapidly in the fluency and reading for meaning needed in Stage 2. This could be dysfunctional for the development of Stage 2, which is characterized by a more fluent, freer approach to reading that relies more heavily on the meaning of the text and the use of content. Too analytic an approach at Stage 2 may hold up silent reading comprehension. (pp. 46–47)

There is considerable research evidence to support the position of Chall and others who advocate the importance of a phonic approach as an initial stage in teaching children to read. An accepted generalization is that normal development in reading ability is associated with skill in transcoding from alphabetic representation to sounds. An associated ability in normal readers is the acquisition of a sight vocabulary that permits meaningful word recognition. However, for dyslexic children who are usually severely delayed and often unable to establish transcoding skills, reading improvement is associated with increases in sight vocabulary. Stanovich (1985), a psychologist and authority on reading, bases his acceptance of this general observation upon his review of the relevant literature and his own studies.

AN ALTERNATE PHONIC APPROACH: THE INITIAL TEACHING ALPHABET

The Initial Teaching Alphabet (i. t. a.) is a recent approach that is intended to regularize the correspondence between letter (character) and sound. The i. t. a. (note the use of lower-case letters) was developed by Sir James Pitman and his associates. Sir James is the grandson of Sir Isaac Pitman, who developed a phonic character system called Phonotypy in the mid-nineteenth century. The i. t. a. is essentially a phonic approach that provides a reliable basis for sounding out a display of "letter" characters. These include letters of the alphabet, some symbols of the International Phonetic Alphabet (I.P.A.), and a few that were devised by Sir James. The symbol-characters of the i. t. a. are presented in Table 3-2. If we compare the i. t. a. characters with those of the I.P.A (Table 1-2), we will note many similarities but also some differences in phonemic values. For example, the Numbers 1 and 44 of the i. t. a. are the same characters, but they stand for different sounds in the two systems.

The basic assumption of the advocates of the i. t. a. is that the inconsistent letter-to-sound correspondence in English spelling is a cause of considerable reading disability. If instruction and readers printed in i. t. a. characters are provided, reading problems, at least for beginners, should be overcome. Early research in the 1960s was carried on in British schools and shortly after in schools in Canada and the United States. The British educator, J. Downing (1967), wrote i. t. a. readers and evaluated some of the results of their use.

Downing considers it necessary to caution us that the i. t. a. should not be regarded as a phonetic alphabet in that it is not designed to be a precise representation of the sounds that an individual makes in speaking English. Rather, the i. t. a. is designed to teach beginning reading throughout the English-speaking world and "for this reason it cannot be expected to reflect regional differences in pronunciation." The i. t. a. "does not signal the speech sounds of the speaker" (Downing, 1967, p. 101).

Some of the findings suggest that if the i. t. a. is used as a first reading and writing system for beginning readers, it will generally produce better results than teaching that employs traditional orthography (t.o.). This holds especially when word recognition is the criterion. However,

TABLE 3-2

THE INITIAL TEACHING ALPHABET (i. t. a)

No.	i.t.a. Character	Name in t.o.[a] Letters	i.t.a. Example	Traditional Spelling
1	æ	ae	ræt	rate
2	b	bee	bi*g*	big
3	c	kee	cat	cat
4	d	dee	do*g*	dog
5	єє	ee	meet	meat
6	f	ef	fill	fill
7	*g*	gae	*g*un	gun
8	h	hae	hat	hat
9	ie	ie	tie	tie
10	j	jae	ji*g*	jig
11	k	kae	kit	kit
12	l	el	lamp	lamp
13	m	em	man	man
14	n	en	net	net
15	œ	œ	tœ	toe
16	p	pee	pig	pig
17	r	rae	run	run
18	s	ess	sad	sad
19	t	tee	tap	tap
20	ue	ue	due	due
21	v	vee	van	van
22	w	wae	will	will
23	y	yae	yell	yell
24	z	zee	zω	zoo
25	ʒ	zess	rœʒ	rose
26	wh	whae	when	when
27	ʧh	chae	ʧhick	chick
28	ʇh	ith	ʇhin	thin
29	ʇh	thee	ʇhen	then
30	ʃh	ish	ʃhip	ship
31	ʒ	zhee	viʒon	vision
32	ŋ	ing	siŋ	sing
33	r	ur	bird	bird
34	ɑ	ah	fɑther	father
35	au	aw	taut	taut
36	a	at	appl	apple
37	e	et	e*gg*	egg
38	i	it	dip	dip
39	o	ot	hot	hot
40	u	ut	u*g*ly	ugly
41	ω	oot	bωk	book
42	ω	oo	mωn	moon
43	ou	ow	vou	vow
44	oi	oi	oil	oil

[a]The letters t.o. stand for traditional orthography.

Note: From *Evaluating the Initial Teaching Alphabet* by J. Downing, 1967, London: Cassell. Reprinted by permission.

when comprehension is the criterion, the difference between i. t. a. and t.o. is minimal and not consistent. There is some indication that slow-learning children and children from underprivileged homes do better with the i. t. a. than with t.o. spellings. Interestingly, the highest achievers—those children who are likely to learn without regard to the approach—showed little or no gain when they started with the i. t. a.

In any event, it should be understood that the Initial Teaching Alphabet is intended as an approach for beginners in reading. It is a transitional approach for the first two and possibly three years of formal school instruction.

Lloyd Dunn and several associates used the i. t. a. approach to teach reading in an experimental study with disadvantaged children in Nashville, Tennessee. The investigators concluded that the i. t. a. stimulated initial reading competence in grade one children. In another American study the i. t. a. was used with first-grade children in Bethlehem, Pennsylvania. The results reported by two teachers in the study (Stewart & Huber, 1966) indicate that the children were able to read "earlier and easier" and experienced the "joy of reading." Although not all of the children progressed at the same rate, each child was able to read independently and with pleasure.

My review of these and several other studies in the United States, Great Britain, and Canada in which the i. t. a. was used as an initial approach to reading suggests the following:

1. The i. t. a. shows a slight advantage over traditional written material for children in the first and second years of schooling.

2. The advantage is somewhat greater for underprivileged children, who presumably had little exposure to books at home, than for the more privileged ones.

3. Spelling was somewhat of a problem. Children taught with traditional writing were on the whole better spellers than children taught with the i. t. a. readers. My assumption is that the transition from i. t. a. readers to traditional written material was responsible for the difference.

4. It may be that whatever advantage the i. t. a. approach has over traditional readers may be in the content rather than the orthography. For the most part, the i. t. a. readers had stories with identifiable plots about children and adults who were more real and interesting than the Dicks and Janes of traditional readers. Teachers as well as children might have enjoyed the new experience.

5. In the light of the foregoing, we can come to no firm conclusion about the efficacy of the i. t. a. as an approach to teaching for all or even most children in the primary grades. There does seem to be an advantage in the use of the i. t. a. with children who have had little exposure to books or to adults who were willing and able to read to them.

As of this writing, the advantages of i. t. a. teaching over other "more traditional" approaches have not been firmly demonstrated in the United States. However, one study followed pupils taught with i. t. a. over an eleven-year period. This study, reported by Mazurkiewicz (1973), concerned 14,000 children in 45 classes in Bethlehem, Pennsylvania. The findings indicate a marked reduction—75 to 80 percent—in children who were in need of remedial reading.

In general, there seems to be more enthusiasm for i. t. a. teaching in Great Britain and Australia than in the United States. It may be that American teachers or their supervisors are less patient in their expectations for statistically significant results than their colleagues abroad. It may also be that differences in populations, in the training of teachers, and in the designs of the studies make for differences in the results. In any event, we should not lose sight of the purpose of the i. t. a. as an initial approach to writing and thus to reading and not as a replacement for traditional orthography in reading materials beyond the third grade at the latest. The British proponents of the i. t. a. emphasize that it is a medium of instruction that can be used with any method, including the phonic and the Look-Say.

LOOK-SAY (THINK)-UNDERSTAND MODELS

However devoted teachers might be to the phonic (sounding-out) approach for the teaching of reading, on the basis of either logic or experience, few would (or should) argue that competence in word-recognition skills is not also essential in learning to read. Roswell and Natchez (1977) sum up a reasonable position:

Competence in word-recognition skills is basic in learning to read. . . . The child needs to learn gradually a variety of strategies: whole-word recognition, sound blending techniques, identification of larger units within words, and how to figure out words through the use of context clues.

On the basis of their experience with improficient readers who had been taught by a method that stressed the learning of letter sounds as the key to the mastery of reading, Roswell and Natchez observe:

Despite the good grasp of basic phonic skills, many of these children could not even handle a pre-primer; because as soon as they met phonically irregular words, their single strategy led to confusion and frustration. . . . Therefore, from the outset, flexibility in word-recognition skills needs to be emphasized. (p. 119)

Before presenting the Look-and-Say Sentence Models, I will direct attention to a number of nonletter (nonverbal) signs that almost everyone would recognize instantly as parts of written materials. The sign & (ampersand) fairly reliably stands for *and*; punctuation marks guide us, but not invariably, to appropriate phrasing; quotation marks, exclamation points, dashes (—), provide other kinds of information that is helpful in the comprehension of text content. When we are engaged in doing arithmetic or higher mathematics, we learn different sets of signs that, like punctuation marks, but much more reliably, provide essential information. However, they have no direct or limited relationship to the sound system of a spoken language. As already noted, ideographs, if verbalized, would evoke a variety of responses from Chinese readers, and still different responses from Japanese and Korean readers.

THE LOOK-SAY-THINK-UNDERSTAND
WORD AND SENTENCE MODELS

Unless a considerable part of what we read is read by sight, we are improficient readers. At the extreme opposite of the phonic approach, if we took the advocates of either literally, is the Look-and-Say Sentence Model. If taken literally, the advocates of Look-and-Say hold that repeated exposure to initially simple texts is all that is required for a child to become familiar with the most frequently used words. However, it is important to appreciate that it is the sentence and not the word that is the meaningful unit of sense. Thus, by reading simple sentences in contexts that have simple words, the child learns to *read for meaning* at the outset. The approach is visual with the underlying assumption that a child can learn to identify graphic shapes (word-forms) as other children taught by the phonic approach sound out the letter sounds. Essentially, the child is exposed to visual language.

Through the use of flash cards and pictures with printed captions and, as soon as possible, with attractive books, children can be expected to learn to read.

Young and Tyre and Roswell and Natchez, among others, recognize that the Look-and-Say and Sentence Model (note my modification to Look-Say (Think)-Understand) is more likely to be successful with children who have been exposed to books and to being read to by adults than with children who are not so privileged. Young and Tyre (1983, p. 48) observe that "Children who are used to being read to and are prepared to guess, find that this is the only introduction they need to reading." Unlike those who are taught by a strict phonic approach, children are encouraged to guess at unfamiliar words, those they have not been taught to sight-read. Guessing, however, is not by mere chance. The "guessed" words must make sense in the context of the particular sentence and the story.

Except for the extremists in the phonic and Look-Say camps, the need for phonic reading is acknowledged, as is the need for a sight vocabulary for the high-frequency words in a language system. In practice, most teachers who are not under a self-imposed or administration-imposed edict to adhere to either approach are likely to employ a combination of methods, adjusting how much they need of each according to the child and his or her proficiency and limitations in reading. This observation holds for other approaches to be described.

The Look-Say Model has had its advocates for many years. It was much in vogue in the 1950s. It still is an approach of choice for many children today.

THE LANGUAGE EXPERIENCE MODEL (LEM)

Both the Phonic Model and the Look-Say Model have an implicit assumption that a preselection of words is necessary to introduce the child to reading. The Phonic Model, at least for English-speaking children, would preselect those words that have a high letter-to-sound (graphemic-phonemic) correspondence. Presumably, this selection will also provide a vocabulary that is initially useful to the child in his or her creative writing efforts. The Look-Say Model is more concerned with words that can be put to use, whether or not they have a graphemic-phonemic correspondence. This model stresses *reading for meaning*.

A very different philosophy and approach are provided in the Language Experience Model (LEM), which may be schematized as:

Child's thought (experience, wishes, fears) → Child's spoken language → Teacher's writing of child's language → Content for reading

The Language Experience Model is associated with Sylvia Ashton-Warner, a New Zealand teacher and novelist. In her book, *Teacher* (1963), Ms. Ashton-Warner explains her philosophy and method, which are based on her experience as a teacher of Maori children. Early in her provocative book, she emphasizes what should constitute a basic vocabulary and content for reading:

First books must be made out of the stuff of the child itself. I reach out into the mind of the child, bring out a handful of the stuff I find there, and use that as our first working material.

★ ★ ★ ★ ★

First words must have an intense meaning for the child. They must be part of his being. . . . They must be words organically tied up, or organically born from the dynamics of life itself.

An obvious advantage of LEM over most other programs is there is no question of meaning related to the choice of words for the initial or key vocabulary. Ashton-Warner does realize that some children and their vocabularies are not readily accessible. For such children, she begins with a General Key Vocabulary, words that she believes are likely to be common to all children in any race or ethnic group. The Key Vocabulary is a number of words bound up with a child's need for security. These include words such as *mummy, daddy, kiss,* and *frightened.* I would add such words as *love, like, hate, good, bad,* and *yucky.* Because the child's language is used, there is no gap between what the child says or might want to say and what the child is taught to read and to write.

The initial approach is to ask the child to draw a picture and to tell about it. If the child cannot or will not draw, he is urged to tell something about an experience. Whether the experience is real or imaginary, the "transformation" from the oral to the written form is shared by the child and the teacher. The written form is, of course, one done by the teacher. The writing may be traced or copied by the child. When it is copied, the child has the beginnings of a book of his own "writing" and certainly of his or her own creation.

This approach, except for deprived children, is not entirely new. Privileged children are often likely to come to school able to write their own names and possibly those of siblings and pets. They may also know how to write *mommy* and *daddy* and a few more words that have special significance for them. Some children have their drawings captioned for them, or do their own captioning from a model. These, of course, are proudly displayed in likely-to-be-seen places so that they may be admired by cooperating friends and relatives. The child who "writes" to dictation on a letter-by-letter basis, or who is able to copy letters, is also exposed to the shape and form of letters, to appropriate sequencing (left to right in English), to punctuation marks, and other characteristics of writing.

A possible limitation of the LEM is in the nature of child language— its early grammatical constructions and paucity of vocabulary. This, of course, pertains only to the initial stages of learning to read. Once the child has passed these stages, the content of instruction should expand the child's vocabulary as well, and, more generally, how to "say" and write a few words well and correctly according to a cultural standard.

The LEM approach is essentially a one-to-one highly motivating experience in learning to read. Soon, however, children are given the opportunity to read their classmates' material. If, with the permission of the child, the material is presented on a chalkboard, the reading becomes a class activity. At the outset, LEM is more time consuming than other approaches to reading. However, the LEM approach may reduce the number of childen who are at high risk for reading failure. Thus, in the long run, time and effort and preventing the frustration of failure may be more financially and emotionally saving than other approaches to reading.

READING AND SPELLING (R-S)

The i. t. a., as already noted, was devised as a method to establish a close correspondence between letter-symbols and sounds for English. The assumption was, and presumably still is, that an "alphabet" with high and consistent letter-to-sound correspondence would make it easier for children to learn to read than the use of traditional orthography. The i. t. a. lent itself readily to phonic approaches to the teaching of reading. However, the notion of teaching spelling together with reading does not necessitate the use of an augmented alphabet to provide for a single letter-symbol to teach reading. Reading and Spelling (R-S) may be taught with traditional orthography and rules that are intended to account for apparent inconsistencies between letters and sounds.

R-S programs are likely to begin with a selected vocabulary of phonically consistent (regular) words that follow phonic reading rules. In essence, through words such as *bit, hit, bat,* and *hat; hot, log, fog;* and *run, fun, sun,* explicit and implicit rules are established that provide the child with insight into the likely pronunciation of words of similar construction. When presented with new words in context, children are directed to sound out the letter presentation and are discouraged from guessing. Spelling is taught along with the phonic transcoding.

Reading and Spelling (R-S) approaches can and should be incorporated into content that provides useful information about syntax and should progress as early as possible into reading for meaning. A limitation of the R-S approach is that there are more than a hundred basic "phonic rules" and many more spellings for which "rules" will be of little help. Without a sight vocabulary, reading is apt to be slow and laborious. The lips as well as moving hands will be involved in writing and often, I have observed, in reading.

For some beginning readers, it may be enough of a challenge and motivation to be able to read single words, phrases, and short sentences, first aloud and then more or less silently, to be involved in the reading game. Other children may be more demanding and insist on material that is interesting. A controlled reading-spelling approach requires creativity on the level of genius to meet such not unreasonable demand.

An interesting adaptation of reading and spelling is provided in a voice recognition system that is a recent development of the IBM Corporation. As described in a Stockholders' Report (2nd quarter, 1986):

The desk-top system features a state-of-the-art microprocessor chip. . . . The chip and associated circuitry make it possible for the Personal Computer A T to use an innovative statistical approach to interpret information entered verbally. The technique breaks each word into a set of phonetic building blocks, then compares the set against the profiles of 5000 words stored in the system and chooses potential matches. As the user continues the sentence, the initial selections are reevaluated in the context in which they are used, and a probable word is selected. This contextual ability enables the system to distinguish between words that sound alike but are spelled differently, such as "no" or "know" and "right" or "write."

It should be noted that the machine and the system have been provided with a knowledge of language so that selections (guesses) of the likely appropriate words are produced. In effect, this IBM voice recognition system is processing spoken language and not just voice. The processing is done with psycholinguistic knowledge incorporated into the system. More of this will be considered in our consideration of psycholinguistics and reading (Chapter Four).

CHAPTER FOUR

Psycholinguistics and Reading

The entire process of reading can best be understood when consideration is given to the devices within language that convey meaning and the ways readers interpret and react to these devices.

★ ★ ★ ★ ★

Understanding how reading works and how children learn language may turn out to be the key to universal literacy.

E. Brooks Smith, Kenneth S. Goodman, and Robert Meredith, *Language and Thinking in School* (1976)

As an identifiable discipline, psycholinguistics includes broad interests that are related to the acquisition of abilities to comprehend and speak a language; the uses of language in human communication; and the study of the different forms and structures employed in efforts to achieve a variety of communicative purposes.

The psychological processes of perception and meaning underlie all aspects of psycholinguistic study. When we speak or when we listen (we learn to listen before we can learn to speak), we are involved with a system or systems—a code or codes if we are bilingual—that presumably relates speech sounds to language that has intended meaning. When we are engaged in reading or in writing, the same implicit assumptions hold for the written code.

Psycholinguistics is a comparatively young discipline. It was born in 1951 when three linguists and three psychologists with a strong interest in language met for a seminar at Cornell University in Ithaca, New York. Their influence has been notable. A recent product of psycholinguistic knowledge and research is an interest in psychological and linguistic processes in reading, with a particular emphasis on reading for meaning.

PSYCHOLINGUISTIC INFLUENCES

Psycholinguists view reading as an *active participatory process* in which the reader is engaged in reconstructing the intended meaning of the author. To accomplish this end, the reader must employ a variety of strategies and relevant cues to arrive at (reconstruct) the writer's meaning. Reading, in common with listening, requires us to make "best guesses" as to the meaning of content and to receive confirmation that these guesses are probably correct. If we receive no confirmation in the process of reading, we can go back and read again, or seek help from a dictionary if we are not certain about, or just do not know, the meaning of a particular word. If this strategy provides confirmation, we go on with our reading. If it does not, we may go back and search for a possible earlier error in comprehension. Reading has an advantage over listening because readers can almost always take a second look at what they have read. Unless we are face-to-face with a friendly speaker, we cannot always ask him or her to repeat or rephrase or explain what was said. For example, in formal lecture situations or when listening to speakers on radio or on television, we must be satisfied, or dissatisfied, with our best guesses as to intended meaning. Talking back may help the listener to feel better, but it will not result in any immediate change of discourse on the part of the speaker.

Psycholinguists provide a psycho-philosophy rather than a specific model or method for teaching reading. Foremost among psycholinguists in their interest and concern about reading are Frank Smith (1973 and 1976) and Kenneth S. Goodman (1976). Like psycholinguists in general, they do not assume that they know all the complex processes, psychological and neurological, that are involved in the process of reading. They do believe, as I do, that children differ in how they learn to read and also in how they read as they mature. They also understand that there are different kinds, styles, and purposes in reading, and with them varying rates and intervals for contemplation. We may read rapidly (skim) to get the gist of a given passage when our interest is in determining its usability for a given purpose. If the material is in keeping with our needs, we may read it a second and even a third time, more slowly and more carefully, for details of information or argument. We may reread rapidly until we arrive at the part of the content for which we were searching. If we are following a recipe or instructions in a do-it-yourself manual, either initially or on a second reading, we are likely to read slowly *one direction at a time.* In general, technical or scientific material is read more slowly and carefully than a newspaper article, a short story, or a novel.

Those who are fond of reading poetry approach different poets with varying attitudes and anticipations. They may read some poetic writings for the sounds and rhythms, others for expressions of emotion, and still others for the imagery and depth of meaning. Students of writing may read to appreciate style, or precision of vocabulary, or clarity and ability to communicate meaning. Other writers, who may be abstruse and possibly profound, may be given slow and considered readings and rereadings. Little of this is taught in the elementary schools and precious little in the secondary grades. Proficient readers learn to do what deserves to be done in the way they approach reading. They do adjust their rate and times for contemplation of meaning in keeping with what they expect to get out of what they read. Some may sound out (phoneticize) when they are reading poetry; some may visualize or do both in keeping with their responses to the material. In contrast, improficient readers seldom make special adjustments to writing, possibly because they have no special or differential expectations in regard to it.

Psycholinguists emphasize that motivation and self-reward are important to keep the reader involved. They also hold that reading is what takes place behind the eyes and between our ears after the reader has taken in the content before his or her eyes. Young and Tyre (1983) sum up what is involved in learning to read and what takes place as we are engaged in reading and in expanding our learning and knowledge of language:

> Learning to read efficiently involves learning to perceive the most significant cues of print as economically as possible. We look for the most significant characteristics of the most significant letters, look for the most meaningful and significant chunks of letters in syllables and words, and look for whole phrases and sentences in one glance. Because we can anticipate from these minimal cues, we are able to read quickly, and hold large chunks of information in memory and access the meaning of what we have read. (p. 54)

Our knowledge and awareness of language, of how words may follow one another in a sequence of writing, of how language is related to thought, help us in the process of reading. A good reader, once involved, begins to anticipate what the text is about and so scans for meaning. If this were not so, if reading were limited to what is before our eyes, that is, to identify and process individual letters or even combinations of letters, our rate of reading would be no greater than 60 words per minute rather than ranging from about 300 to up to 1,000 words for persons who can do speed reading.

Following are a few "exercises" to test anticipation in reading. The same anticipation (expectancy) would, of course, hold for listening.

Last weekend the weather was fair on Saturday, but it _ _ _ _ _ _ on _ _ _ _ _ _.

Up and _ _ _ _ Tim and Mary _ _ _ _ on the teeter-_ _ _ _ _ _.

Lewis Carroll's famous *Jabberwocky* presents a different kind of psycholinguistic challenge to arrive at tentative meaning.

> 'Twas brillig, and the slithy toves
> Did gyre and gimble in the wabe;
> All mimsy were the borogoves,
> And the mome raths outgrabe.

Knowing that this excerpt comes from *Through the Looking Glass* helps us to decide that it is nonsense verse, and that we need not try to arrive at any precise meaning. But we are able to guess at possible meanings. For instance, we would guess that *brillig* is a verb or an adjective because it follows' 'twas (it was); because of its position at the end of the line, following an earlier verb-phrase ('twas brillig), we anticipate a noun phrase, and so assign adjective (attribute) significance to *slithy* and nominal significance to *toves*. Because *toves* ends with an *s*, we assume that whatever a *tove* might be, there are more than one of the creatures. Other meanings might be guessed at because of their resemblance to words that we know. Function words such as *and, the, to, for* (articles, auxiliary verbs, prepositions, and conjunctions—the small words of conventional grammar) help us to guess at the likely grammatical construction and so to arrive at meaning. For *Jabberwocky* this would be:

> 'Twas .... and the ....
> Did .... and ...... in the ....;
> All ..... were the ....,
> And the ....

Incidentally, would the number of dots and the spacing help the reader guess at the possible words?

In general, we can also anticipate that a sentence that begins with the word "Although" is likely to be longer and more complex than one beginning with "Joe is a" or one with "Who," "When," or "Where" as the initial word.

It should now be apparent that to read proficiently, one must have not only a knowledge of language but experiences of the world that may be encoded into language. In classroom situations beginning in the early grades, the teacher's task is to provide and share relevant experiences, direct and vicarious, with the pupils. Children themselves must share experiences with their classmates. This is the essence of the Language Experience Model described in Chapter Three.

When engaged in reading a language that employs alphabetic symbols, among other things, the reader must learn whether to scan from left to right, as in Western languages, or right to left, as in Hebrew and Arabic. For English-speaking readers, reading then becomes a process of scanning from left to right the units of language that are encoded in alphabetic symbols so that the symbols are decoded in the contexts in which they are presented. Usually, readers apprehend meaning in the sentence-by-sentence presentations. Sometimes, by design, the meaning of a passage does not become evident until the last sentence or, possibly, the last phrase of a passage has been read. For example, consider the passage that follows:

Jones had an unusual work history. Somehow, he managed to get himself fired at least once a week. But not until his last firing, when he was seriously injured, did Jones decide to give up his career as a human cannonball.

Few children who are beginning their own careers as readers are likely to have either the experience or psycholinguistic knowledge to understand this passage. But some may. For the present, let us return to how to establish knowledge and motivate the child to want to learn to read. The suggestions that follow are for the parent, if the child is not resistant, and for the primary grade teacher who is responsible for getting the child on his or her way to becoming "hooked" on reading. The suggestions are adaptations of "Twelve Easy Ways of Making Learning to Read Easy" offered by Peter Young and Colin Tyre in their book *Dyslexia or Illiteracy?* (1983, p. 57).

1. On as regular a basis as possible, read aloud books and selected materials from children's magazines that will involve the child in an enjoyable listening experience. If the child is ready and not chronically "antsy," he or she should become motivated to wish to learn to read.

2. In early reading sessions, move your finger under each line of print so that the child develops left-to-right eye scanning. Later, it should be enough for you to place a finger to the left of each line as a guide to where you are in the reading.

3. Talk to and with the child about what you are going to read and later—child willing—about what you have read. This should help both of you to learn whether the child understood, or on what level there was understanding. It should also help to make the child aware of language in print and the need for attentive listening.

4. As soon as possible, get the child to read with you in unison. This "choral" (supported) reading should help the child to become "print-borne."

5. To develop language awareness, play word games such as rhyming, finishing phrases or sentences, I Spy, Hangman, or charades.

6. To develop skills in sequencing and in memory, build up an inventory of favorite rhymes and jingles, of songs and jokes, which the child enjoys and learns by heart. These may be printed on cards for the child to use as prompts in his or her own reading.

7. When you read aloud to the child, encourage guessing as to what comes next when you pause intentionally. If what the child offers is not in the material you are reading but makes sense in light of the context, congratulate the child on the effort. Then you may say, "Here is how the author wrote it" and read the writer's version.

8. To help establish selective attention, use the material you are reading to play "Find the word that says . . . ; "Find the word that begins with . . . ; "Find the word that ends with . . . ." For a sophisticated child, you might try, "Find the word that rhymes with. . . ." This game should enhance the child's awareness of language and, on a visual-perceptual level, some of the patterns and characteristics of printed forms.

9. When you are confident that the child has some reading ability, you may ask the child to read sentences or short passages that were first read in unison. Young and Tyre refer to this as "prepared reading." On occasion, you might exchange roles with the child to give him or her a sense of verbal power and control.

10. Praise the child for his or her effort, for attention and evidence of increased attention.

11. If the child is uncertain about a correct response, encourage guessing. If the child is unwilling to guess or has guessed wrong, offer the correct response before he or she becomes anxious. "A little and often is better than a lot rarely."

12. Reading should be fun! Do all you can to make it so.

The twelve "easy ways" are not to be regarded as "how to's" or as a hierarchy of steps or stages. The teacher's responsibility is to apply them, with individual adaptation, to each child in light of the child's interests and readiness for motivation. Where and when to begin will depend on the teacher's appreciation of the child as a personality, and an assessment, formal or informal, of what the child knows about language. Perhaps, above all, the determining factor may be what the teacher knows about how the child is best at learning.

Where to begin (which suggestion to follow first) is also an individual matter. It is probably better to begin at a level at which a child is almost sure to be successful than to risk a level at which a child may experience failure. The likelihood that reading will be an enjoyable undertaking and an accomplishment is enhanced by success. Even small successes are better than small failures. In the minds of many children, there are no small failures. This is especially so in the minds of anxious children!

IMPROFICIENT READERS AND KNOWLEDGE OF LANGUAGE

This discussion will be limited to readers, children in the primary and secondary grades, who are improficient in their comprehension of written language, but are not dyslexic. (Dyslexia, a severe reading deficiency, and its likely causes, will be considered in Chapters Six and Seven.) The children with whom we will be concerned in this discussion are presumably of normal or above-normal intelligence and are without significant sensory, motor, or emotional impairment. Again, presumably, their academic achievements are within the normal range of expectation. (I say presumably, because I speculate that were the children better readers, they might also be better achievers.)

A general observation, based on recent research, is that improficient readers are likely to have some degree of language deficiency. Sometimes these deficiencies are subtle and not readily detectable. In some instances, the deficiencies become more readily apparent and are revealed in word-finding difficulty or in misuse of words. In other instances, grammatical inadequacies become evident in writing. Generally, improficient readers exhibit inadequacy in over-all verbal learning. For children whose language difficulties range from mild to moderately severe, the term *specific reading disability* is often applied. The most severely impaired may be identified as *probable dyslexics* or *dyslexics*.

An excellent and fairly detailed review of the literature by Vellutino (1983) is the basis for the following general observations about improficient readers considered as a total, "special" population.

Poor readers are less able than proficient readers to identify and arrive at the meaning of abstract words. They do better with concrete words. The weakness with the abstract carries over to identifying and knowing the meaning of prefix and suffix constructions. These are abstract grammatical markers that modify the meaning of basic root words. These grammatical markers are used to designate number, gender, person, case, and tense. Except in dialects in which the conventional use of grammatical markers may not be observed, a lack of knowledge or lack of sensitivity to the functions of grammatical markers interferes with an adequate decoding of spoken as well as written language. By the age of nine or ten, almost all children somehow (rarely by direct teaching) acquire their knowledge of the rules that govern sentence construction. These include basic syntax and their knowledge of how to understand and use grammatical markers that have no meaning except when they are affixed to root syllables. Thus they have no difficulty in decoding and understanding the difference between "Mary is walking to school," "Mary likes to walk," and "Yesterday, because it was raining, Mary did not walk to school."

Another general observation is that improficient readers have inadequate vocabularies both in terms of the number of words they know and the meanings of the words they seem to know. Because many words have several possible meanings, the specific likely meaning can be determined only in context. Thus, improficient readers are more likely than good readers to make errors in arriving at the meanings of *run* in "Run up the flag" and "Run up the stairs," as well as "Tom is run down" and "Tom was run down." The last example is ambiguous unless we have some information about Tom's health or his involvement in an accident.

Sentences such as "Tom told Bill he's going to the movies," or "John told his brother Bob he must swim" are also likely to be misunderstood. An assumption (rule) that improficient readers seem to follow is that the noun or pronoun that is closest to the final verb phrase (in the example above, *to swim*) is the subject of that phrase; thus they would conclude that Bill is going to the movies or that Bob is the one who must swim.

Vellutino, the expert and investigator on reading and children with reading problems (cited above), sums up his findings about poor readers by noting that: "There is now much evidence that poor readers are hampered by substantial difficulties in semantic processing which appear to be associated with specific problems in word encoding and retrieval as well as with deficiencies in lexical development" (1983, p. 157). In addition, as I have noted, their syntactic (grammatical) knowledge may also be deficient.

The implications of these observations are that instruction in writing and reading should not end with the elementary school grades. Instruction for many children, and especially for those who had early difficulties in learning to read for meaning, should continue throughout the secondary grades. Such instruction needs to include development of vocabulary that may express nuances of meaning and feeling, the writing and understanding of sentences that are necessarily complex, and, above all, if possible by teacher example, an appreciation of and sensitivity to well-spoken or well-written language. Chapter Eleven deals with levels and types of instruction in reading that are not usually taught in our public schools.

CHAPTER FIVE

The Brain, Language, and Reading

We happen to live in a society in which the child who has trouble learning to read is in difficulty. Yet we have all seen some dyslexic children who draw much better than controls, i.e., who have either superior visual-perceptual or visual-motor skills. My suspicion would be that in an illiterate society such a child would be in little difficulty and might, in fact, do better because of his visual-perceptual talents, while many of us who function well here might do poorly in a society in which quite a different array of talents was needed to be successful.

Norman Geschwind (1979)

Comparing the human brain to a computer is an intriguing but misleading analogy. The brain is composed of living tissue; so it can grow and change without outside intervention. The computer does not have this potential. Again, although it is tempting to compare the nerve cells (neurons) of the brain and their complex of interconnections to a computer's "wiring" system, the analogy is misleading. Ornstein and Thompson (1984, p. 61) explain that "a neuron is not simply (either) on or off like an element in a computer; it is always processing the information it receives from thousands of other nerve cells and from chemical messengers . . . and is always communicating with many other nerve cells."

The complexity of the brain, and the many billions of nerve cells—perhaps as many as 100 billion in the brain as a whole—that are responsible for receiving and transmitting information should give one pause before attempting a cut-and-dried explanation of how the brain deals with language, spoken or written. With this reservation in mind, the reader is cautioned to consider everything that follows tentatively. What follows is, however, based on findings that I consider to be authoritative and to represent the present state of knowledge on brain and language functioning.

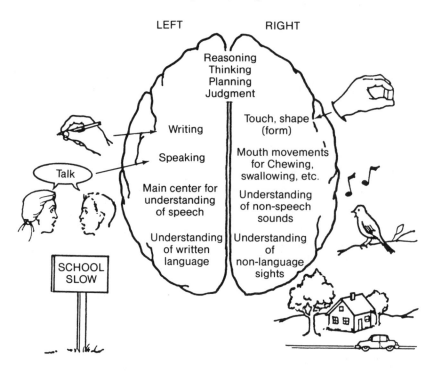

FIGURE 5–1. The cortex of the brain showing differential functions within the hemisphere and between the left and right hemispheres. Reflexive nonspeech movements as in chewing, sucking, swallowing, and nonlanguage mouth noises are controlled by centers in the lower brain. These centers have connections with the indicated area in the right hemisphere. For speech, both the left and right hemispheres are involved; the left, Broca's area, usually is dominant.

THE INDIVIDUAL AND INDIVIDUALIZED BRAIN

Brains are "constructed" and organized according to a common pattern (see diagram of the brain cortex, Figure 5-1), *but no two brains are exactly the same.* One person's brain may have larger "bulges" in one area than do most other persons, and smaller than average "bulges" in others. One human brain may have a larger than "normal" occipital lobe (the area in the back portion of the cortex that processes visual information) and a smaller than normal temporal lobe (the area that deals with auditory information). With such individual variations, we should expect differences in how given brains function, and so, perhaps, understand why some persons are strongly ear-minded, others visually minded, and still others motor-minded. Those who are strongly motor-minded need to experience how speech sounds are produced—to be aware of their articulatory movements—so that they may feel confident about what they say and hear.

Human brains are individually different. This is so because brains at birth may have variations of a common pattern and also because human beings, brains included, are remarkably immature at birth. As brains develop, they are influenced by the individual's interactions with the outside world. Thus brains are impressed according to individual experiences as their possessors mature as persons and personalities.

CEREBRAL LATERALITY (DOMINANCE) AND LANGUAGE

The entire brain is divided into two halves or hemispheres. Until fairly recently the hemispheres were considered to be identical in structure but known to be different in function. Beginning in the 1950s, structural differences were discovered that presumably account for some of the differences in function. Figure 5-1 of the brain cortex, the outer layer of the brain, indicates some of the differences in function with special attention given to spoken and written language.

For almost all right-handed persons and about 60 to 70 percent of the left-handed, the left hemisphere is normally the one that deals with—processes—language, spoken or written. But the right hemisphere is neither deaf nor mute. The subordinate hemisphere, though not dominant for language, is normally dominant for the processing of music, for environmental nonspeech sounds, and probably even for human nonspeech noises. It is likely that when we learn to sing a song, the right hemisphere processes the melody while the left hemisphere learns the words.

Specifically, for most of us, the left auditory area (Main Center for understanding speech in Figure 5-1) is necessary for speech processing, and the analogous right hemisphere region is the processor for nonspeech sounds. Visual intake is differentiated along the same line. The left visual area—the posterior portion of the brain cortex—is normally concerned with the comprehension of written language, while the right cortical area processes nonlanguage events.

Farther front in the brain cortex is the area for control of movement. In regard to language, as our diagram (Figure 5-1) indicates, the left hemisphere has an area that controls movements for speaking (articulation) and writing. The corresponding right cortical area in association with lower brain centers normally controls movements involved with chewing, swallowing, and other nonlanguage behaviors. Still farther front, the anterior portion of the brain (the frontal lobes), is the center for reasoning, thinking, judgment, and planning.

Again, what I have just described is a general plan of structure and functional organization and especially for cerebral dominance for language, spoken and written. There are numerous individual exceptions. Most occur along the following lines as they relate to dominance for language.

HANDEDNESS AND BRAIN DOMINANCE FOR LANGUAGE

Upward of 95 percent of right-handed persons have cerebral dominance for language in the left hemisphere. Thus, we have an "exceptional" right-handed population of from 1 to 5 percent who have language dominance in the right rather than the left hemisphere.

About 60 percent of the left-handed also have language dominance in the left hemisphere. However, the degree of dominance (left over right) is not as strong as it is with the vast majority of the right-handed. The other 40 percent of the left-handed have right hemisphere dominance for language, but, as with the first group, the degree of dominance is not as strong as with the nonexceptional right-handed.

Ambidextrous persons follow the pattern of the left-handed. There is also a small population who are ambinondextrous (equally awkward and unskilled with either hand) who probably have no clear dominance for language as well as for motor functions. This population, less than 1 percent, tends to have "scribble" speech and illegible writing. The family background of this small but challenging population reveals members, mostly males, with similar speech and language problems, including reading and writing. The left-handed constitute about 10 percent of the total population. As a special subpopulation, they do not follow the general pattern of having language dominance in the hemisphere contralateral to their expressed handedness. One way of explaining this deviation is the possibility that the language functions of the left-handed are more widely dispersed in both hemispheres of the brain than they are with 95 percent or more of the right-handed. Support for this assumption is the substantial information that left-handed persons, children as well as adults, recover from language disruptions and deficits resulting from brain damage earlier and better than do the right-handed. However, children below age 12, presumably because of the plasticity of their brains, show better recovery from the effects of brain damage than adolescents and adults.

Some brains do organize differently from the common pattern. In some instances, the atypical organization may be congenital. In other instances, it may be as a result of early brain damage. Atypical organization may also be a consequence of circumstances and learning experiences that may promote the development of function in one area of the brain at the possible expense of other areas. For instance, a parent or preschool teacher who is strongly visually minded may emphasize this modality intake and deemphasize the auditory. Thus, a child may develop a greater than normal inclination for visual intake and a lesser one for the auditory.

Brains, especially young ones, also have a capacity for reorganization in the event of disease or injury. In some instances, brain dominance may be shifted from one hemisphere—normally genetic—to the other for which it was not normally or initially dominant. We might also conjecture that left-handed persons and ambidextrous persons do not lose cortical plasticity as they grow older and so have less difficulty than the right-handed in shifting cerebral dominance. This observation may account for the good recovery for language function in the left-handed and ambidextrous compared with the right-handed after incurring brain damage. For more detailed discussions of cerebral dominance and language see Eisenson (1986, Chapter 7) and Springer and Deutsch (1981).

THE FOREBRAIN AND LANGUAGE PLANNING

We shall return to brain organization and cerebral dominance for language in a later consideration of dyslexia. Here I will present my view of the role of the forebrain of the cortex for language functioning, particularly with regard to what the consequences are likely to be if the forebrain is either retarded in development or injured by accident or disease.

The anterior part of the brain is proportionately much larger in human beings than in any other primates. This area, as noted earlier (Figure 5-1), is concerned with planning, judgment, and reasoning. These high-level cognitive functions are associated with language and thinking.

Every spoken utterance requires, pre-formulation (What shall I say? and How shall I say it?) for the organization of a planned sequence of sounds into words, specifically words that are selected for the occasion and arranged into conventional (grammatic) utterances. For writing, an analogous plan must be entertained and produced. This plan will include the sequence of the letters for the words, and the words into conventional written constructions. The rules for writing are considerably stricter than the rules for speaking, which, unless memorized, may include incomplete sentences and agrammatic constructions.

BRAIN DAMAGE AND LANGUAGE IMPAIRMENT

Now, what may the language consequences be if the anterior area of the brain is underdeveloped, or damaged as a result of disease or injury? For damaged brains in young children—below age 9—there is a disruption of language functioning. The period of disruption, if only one hemisphere of the brain is damaged, is usually followed by rapid recovery, but possibly not by complete restoration of all language functions. With congenitally underdeveloped brains (maturational delay) there is likely to be significant retardation in language production and later for reading and writing.

Other specialized areas of the brain concerned with language must, of course, be in constant communication with the forebrain so that the linguistic plan may be carried out. This holds from the time of initial intake through seeing or hearing to its potential and then actual execution in speech or writing. We may note from Figures 5-1 and 5-2 that the specialized intake areas that deal with language are in the posterior portion of the brain cortex and the output areas are in the front portion of the brain. Damage to any of these areas of the left hemisphere in the vast majority of the right-handed almost always produces an initial disruption of one or more language functions. Recovery, as already indicated, takes place more easily for young persons than for the adolescent and post-adolescent population. Damage to the posterior portion of the brain may impair reading comprehension. This would constitute an acquired dyslexia for those who were able to read. For reasons previously explained, the left-handed and the ambidextrous, even though they too experience initial disruptions in language, have a better rate and degree of recovery.

Children who incur brain damage either before birth or during the birth process are at high risk for being delayed and impaired in acquiring language. Children who have slow maturation of the critical language centers, either for intake or output, are very likely to be delayed in learning to speak. If the damage is to the auditory area, their impairments may be for understanding speech and so, without understanding, also for speech production. Depending upon degree of impairment, these children would be designated as dysphasic (mild to moderate degree), or aphasic if more severe. This population of children who are at high risk for reading difficulty and for writing are included in the category of the dyslexic.

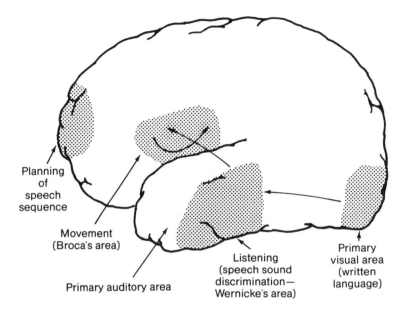

Planning
of
speech
sequence

Movement
(Broca's area)

Primary auditory area

Listening
(speech sound
discrimination—
Wernicke's area)

Primary
visual area
(written
language)

FIGURE 5–2. Projections of neural circuitry when a person hears spoken language and processes the content by repeating it and then decoding it for meaning. According to my speculation, the spoken content is heard in the primary auditory area and is analyzed for its speech sound content in Wernicke's area. If the listener decides to speak (repeat) the word or words he or she hears, the messages are first transmitted to the frontal area for an appropriate speech plan, then to Broca's area for the execution of the plan. Monitoring, as shown in the plan in the figure above, takes place by feedback to Wernicke's area to ascertain whether the repetition of the spoken content is correct. Adapted from "Specialization of the Human Brain," by Norman Geschwind, in *The Brain* (p. 113), 1979, San Francisco: W. H. Freeman and Company.

BRAIN AND LANGUAGE: THE PRESENT STATE OF KNOWLEDGE

It would be unfair to the reader to pretend that the explanations offered in the previous pages are entirely adequate and tell us all that we need to know about the relationship of the brain to the human species specific behavior we call language. We are, in fact, just beginning to discover what might take place not only in the brain but throughout the entire neurological system when, first as infants and then as adults, we learn to understand spoken language and learn to speak. The processes involved in learning to read have their own complexities about which we can make educated conjectures, but we should not pretend that we are dealing with certainties.

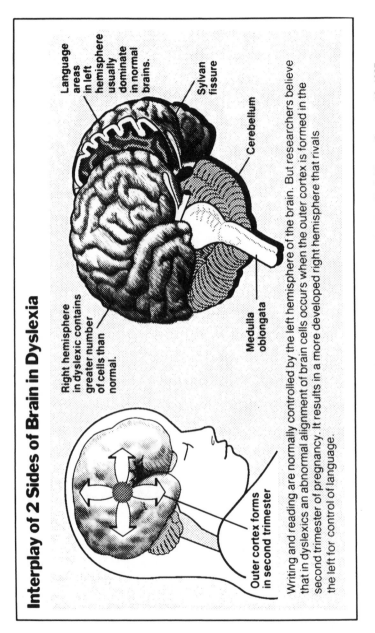

FIGURE 5–3. A speculative explanation of brain differences in dyslexics. From *The New York Times*, January 13, 1987. Reprinted by permission.

The available neurological literature provides many exceptions to the observations about the general plan for learning to speak and to read and to write. On the other hand, there is considerable evidence to support the general observations relative to the functional differences between the hemispheres and to the concept of cerebral dominance for language. Unfortunately, because so much of the evidence to date comes to us from autopsy findings of brains damaged by disease or injury, we have been gathering our data from atypical populations.

The future may be brighter for obtaining the information we need about the neurology and neuropathology of spoken and written language. The sophisticated instrumentation that is now becoming available should enable us to obtain information and insights into normal brain functioning as well as what goes awry with abnormal brains. Without being limited by autopsy findings, we will have a variety of populations for study. These populations will include children, adolescents, and adults, normal speakers and readers, and those who are improficient in either or both speaking and reading.

BRAIN DIFFERENCES IN DYSLEXICS

Recent research evidence at the Children's Hospital and Beth Israel Hospital in Boston (Galaburda, 1985) provides a speculative position as to likely brain differences in dyslexics. According to the observations of researchers at these hospitals, the dyslexic child may have suffered subtle brain damage in the fetal stage of development with resultant variations in cellular brain structure. A significant variation is an increase over the usual number of cells in the right hemisphere at the expense of the left. Specifically, the language areas of the right hemisphere are as large as those of the left. Therefore, at least theoretically, the two hemispheres of the brain become rivals for the control of reading and writing as well as other, earlier established, language functions. Figure 5-3 is a diagrammatic representation of what may occur in the brain of dyslexics.

With these observations and reservations, in the next chapters I will undertake to explain the nature of the severe reading problems identified collectively as dyslexia and the subtypes of dyslexia. Included will be an explanation of why more Johnnies than Joannies are likely to be dyslexic. As a closing note to this chapter we should note the observation of research neurologist Dr. Albert Galaburda (1985), who says that the evidence of recent research indicates that:

. . . dyslexics often have important talents in the visual arts, athletics, music, and mathematics. Failure to insure adequate remediation therefore means that not only does the individual dyslexic fail to achieve his full potential but also that the society is deprived of the services of highly talented individuals.

We will return to this observation in Chapter Eight, in which we consider "Dyslexia in Persons of Eminence."

CHAPTER SIX

The Syndrome of Dyslexia

I was unfitted for school work. I had to give the whole evening
to one lesson if I was to know it. . . . My thoughts were a
great excitement, but when I tried to do anything with them,
it was like trying to pack a balloon into a shed in a high wind. I
was always near the bottom of my class, and always making
excuses that but added to my timidity.

William Butler Yeats, *Autobiographies* (1926)

In the first chapter dyslexia was defined as a severe disability of children
to learn to read that is not acounted for by emotional factors, or intellectual limitations, or lack of opportunity for instruction. It was also noted
that dyslexic children almost always follow a familial pattern that
includes members with learning disabilities and that the incidence
includes three to four times as many boys as girls. The familial pattern
and the male to female ratio strongly suggest a genetic basis for dyslexia.

A syndrome, as we know, is a complex of symptoms that differentiates
one physiological condition or a medical condition from another. In
medicine, a syndrome refers to disease or pathology. Dyslexia is not a
disease, but it is a condition that needs to be differentiated from others
with which it may share individual symptoms. Is there an identifiable
syndrome that can cause a child to fail to learn to read, or make the
learning of reading exceedingly difficult and at best result in improficient reading? Is there an entity that we can with confidence diagnose as
constitutional dyslexia? I think there is, but some authorities have
reservations. For example, Smith, Goodman, and Meredith state that
"Research has failed to find any substantial cause for reading failure in
physical, mental, or perceptual difficulties" (Goodman et al., 1976, p.
279).

Vellutino (1979, pp. 354–355) is not as firm in his position as are
Goodman and his associates about possible neurophysiological cause or
causes of dyslexia. Vellutino observes that:

Although it may be reasonable that specific types of reading disorder may be linked to different antecedent conditions, given the complexities of this process, it does not seem reasonable to assume that each of these deficiencies is associated with a particular neurological syndrome. Nor is it likely that dysfunction in any one of the sensory or motor systems typically involved in reading (vision, language, speech-motor articulation) necessarily results in reading disability.

Vellutino (1979, 1987) appears to admit that there is a syndrome of dyslexia that has its basis or cause in genetic neurological deviancy. However, he does not see the need for assuming that the variety of deficiencies that accompany dyslexia require separate neurological explanations. Nor can we deny that there are children who despite visual, speech-motor, and to some degree, even language problems, are able to learn to read. We can, of course, speculate that without these sensory-motor and language deficiencies these children might be better readers than we find them to be.

My own position is close to that of the neurologist, Martha B. Dencla, who is professionally concerned with children with learning disabilities and with the "specific" disability of dyslexia. Dencla (1977, p. 29) states: "When we use the term *dyslexia*, we are intending to implicate the *brain* in the chain or network of causation underlying reading disability."

DIFFERENTIAL SYNDROMES

Following are some positions that describe separate and presumably differential *syndromes of dyslexias*. These are based on observations of types of difficulties (errors) made by persons with severe reading problems and errors made in writing.

Boder (1973), a pediatric neurologist, holds that developmentally dyslexic children may be subdivided into three groups according to the patterns of errors they produce in reading and spelling. One group, the "visually impaired," whom Boder designates as the *dyseidetic*, have difficulty in learning to read by a whole-word approach. Dyseidetic children make frequent letter reversal errors such as *no* for *on*, *saw* for *was*, *pan* for *nap*, and *pest* for *step*. Apparently these deficient readers who show evidence of visual discrimination and sequencing errors are not guided by the meaning of the over-all context in the decoding of single words. Spelling errors parallel those for reading, with "phonetic" mistakes (letter for sound) predominating.

The children in Boder's second subgroup show evidence of auditory impairments and are designated as *dysphonetics*. Deficient in phonetic analysis, they are less analytical and more global in reading than dyseidetics. These children would have considerable difficulty in learning to read by a "phonetic" (phonemic) approach and theoretically at least, should be able to learn to read by a whole-word (look-say-think-understand) model.

Boder's third and largest group shows evidence of both visual and auditory deficits; these children show deficiencies that characterize both the dyseidetic and dysphonetic children.

Vellutino (1979), a critic of Boder's position, argues that improper teaching rather than an underlying neurological disorder may account for the described reading difficulties. Specifically, a child may fail to become a proficient reader as a result of being taught exclusively by either a look-say or sounding out (phonemic) approach. However, a study by Rozin and associates (1971) provides evidence that some children who could not learn to read by a phonemic method were able to learn through a "whole word" look-say-understand approach. In this study, eight second-grade children from a Philadelphia "inner city" school who were unable to learn to read by a phonemic approach (letter to sound correspondence) were individually instructed to assign English words to 30 Chinese characters. Within two and a half to five and a half hours, the children learned the task. That is, they spoke an appropriate English word for a Chinese character—an ideogram. The children were also able to arrange the Chinese characters into sentences that followed left to right conventional word order and so produce the equivalent of acceptable English sentences with non-English symbols.

Even if we allow for the novelty of the teaching situation and for motivation in the one-to-one tutorial relationship, the implications of the study must be taken seriously. A selected group of children who were failing to learn to read by one approach—the phonemic—were able to learn by an alternative method that assigned meaning to a graphic presentation on a word level. This approach may have been effective because it bypassed an inefficient intake system that required auditory analysis and appealed directly to a visual system that was ready for the task of decoding written representations on the whole word level.

Pirozzolo, in his *Neuropsychology of Developmental Reading Disorders* (1979), has two broad categories of dyslexia much along the line of Boder's. The children in one category, the *auditory-dyslexic*, have difficulty in over-all language learning and in related problems that are comparable to those of Boder's *dysphonetic* children. The second category, the *visual-spatial* dyslexic children, have difficulties in visual discrimination and letter (sound) sequencing that are comparable to those of Boder's *dyseidetic* group.

In his book Pirozzolo provides research evidence to support his two dyslexic categories. Most of the research compares children who are proficient in reading with dyslexic children on eye movement studies while engaged in reading. On the basis of his findings and other research in the published literature, Pirozzolo conjectures that delayed maturation of nerve fiber pathways is responsible for the reading deficits.

A maturational lag implies a potential for catching up rather than a permanent structural and related functional impairment. If the "catching up" is even and not too long in time, a child may learn to read beginning at age nine or ten despite severe difficulty in earlier years. If the child is not "turned off" and convinced that he or she will forever be a nonreader, the child may still learn to read. Indeed, this happily is the case in many instances in public and perhaps more often in private school settings. As earlier indicated, this "catching up" may explain the low rate of reading difficulty in Russia and the schools in the Scandinavian countries in which formal teaching of reading is not initiated until age seven and sometimes intentionally delayed until age eight or later for the child who is unresponsive to reading.

The possibility that the brain and particularly the centers that are involved in reading continue to mature well beyond adolescence may account for some "miraculous instances" of dyslexics who "suddenly" learned to read while in the secondary grades. There is little question that cerebral maturation continues at least until 30 years of age and possibly into the fourth and fifth decades of life. Maturation is associated with the process of myelinization, which insulates nerve fibers and enhances the conduction and transmission of impulses in the central nervous system. (See Norton, 1975, for a technical discussion of cerebral maturation.)

In *The Dyslexic Child* (1970), Dr. Macdonald Critchley, the British neurologist and president of the World Federation of Neurology, sums up his impressions and the implications of the maturational lag hypothesis.

This attractive hypothesis raises certain questions. If specific developmental dyslexia represents a peculiar type of cerebral immaturity, it follows that the difficulty in reading might eventually improve—provided, of course, that attempts to learn are continued long enough. . . . But of course the opportunities for learning slip by all too quickly. More information is needed here. Developmental dyslexia is certainly not often diagnosed in adulthood even though genuine instances are encountered from time to time. One naturally asks why they should be so uncommon. Perhaps the patient and his parents have resigned themselves to a state of hopeless ineducability, and no longer importune doctors and teachers. The victims may have merged into the amorphous population of adult illiterates and semi-illiterates. Maybe he has eventually made such improvement as to achieve modest social and economic adjustment, but remains a poor speller, an unwilling correspondent, and a reluctant reader. Finally, it is conceivable that the childhood dyslexic—the slow bloomer— eventually matures and blossoms, so as no longer to be conspicuously handicapped. . . .

The cerebral activity which lags behind in maturation may be a specific cognitive act in which verbal symbols, acoustic as well as visual, fail to achieve identity. (Critchley, 1970, pp. 105–106)

In keeping with their view of the disorder, Critchley and Critchley (1978) provide a definition of developmental dyslexia as:

A learning-disability which initially shows itself by difficulty in learning to read, and later by erratic spelling and by lack of facility in manipulating written as opposed to spoken words. The condition is cognitive in essence, and usually genetically determined. It is not due to intellectual inadequacy or to lack of socio-cultural opportunity, or to faults in the technique of teaching, or to emotional factors, or to any known structural brain-defect. It probably represents a specific maturational defect which tends to lessen as the child grows older, and is capable of considerable improvement, especially when appropriate remedial help is afforded at the earliest opportunity (p. 149).

Cognitive processes include perception, concept formation, thinking, memory, learning (including learning how we learn), problem solving, and of course, language acquisition and expression in all of their aspects and modes. Reading is a cognitive process because of its inherent relationship to language. Reading is also a cognitive process because when we are decoding to arrive at meaning, we are engaged in problem solving.

The last of the classification systems that we shall consider is based on a study by Mattis, French, and Rapin (1975) and their review of the related literature. Drs. Mattis, French, and Rapin are members of the Department of Neurology (Division of Neuropsychology) of the Montefiore Hospital and Medical Center in New York City. The children in their study had been referred by pediatric neurologists for learning and behavior disorders. The subjects of the study ranged in age from 8 to 18, were found to have estimated IQs of 80 or above (low normal or above), and normal vision and hearing. Further, those selected for the study showed "no evidence of psychosis or thought disorder." In addition, despite their reading problems, all "had adequate academic exposure." Mattis and his associates identified three clusters of disorders, which they believe account for at least 90 percent of dyslexic and associated impairments.

On the basis of psychological, neurological, and neuropsychological testing, the three groups were identified along the following lines:

1. *Language Disorder Group:* Thirty-nine percent of the subjects fell into this category. Their deficiencies included naming, comprehension of spoken directions, errors in imitative speech, and disorders in speech sound discrimination.

2. *Articulation and Graphomotor Disorders:* The children in this category, about 37 percent, had difficulty in sound-blending and copying of geometric figures and designs. Comprehension of spoken language was adequate.

3. *Visual Perception Disorders:* About 16 percent of the children fell into this category. These subjects had difficulty in remembering and reproducing designs and in organizing design patterns. Their scores were significantly below expectations projected from IQs. They had no apparent difficulty in spoken language comprehension. The details of the evaluations are provided in Mattis, French, & Rapin (1975).

These cluster-categories reveal both similarities and differences, with the greatest overlap in the language and articulation groups. This is not surprising because recent studies have found that children with severe articulation disorders, going beyond lisping and *r*, *l*, *w* substitutions, are also likely to be delayed in language development. The reverse is also found; that is, children who are significantly delayed in language development are also likely to have more than the usual amount of infantile articulation patterns. I review the relationship between disorders of articulation and language delay and disorders in Chapter 7 of *Aphasia and Related Disorders* (1984).

In effect, children who maintain deviant articulation so that their pronunciations are often unintelligible, or who continue to substitute sounds such as *f* for *s*, or who omit syllables such as *tephone* for *telephone*, or who simplify sound blends and produce *poon* for *spoon* beyond the age of "normal" infantile speech should be suspect of also being delayed in overall language development. Research has found this to be so. It is therefore not surprising that children with reading problems often have underlying language deficiencies. They are also most likely to have related learning problems. This observation is supported by our information that the children in the Mattis, French, and Rapin study were referred to the investigators because they had *learning* as well as behavior problems.

LANGUAGE, LEARNING, AND READING DISABILITIES

It should be obvious that a child who has a reading disability will have difficulty in learning what the schools undertake to teach. This is increasingly so beyond the third grade when learning requires the ability to read for comprehension of content, regardless of the subject matter. Is the child who cannot read for compehension one who has a *specific learning disability*? The close relationship between the two is recognized by the legal definition in the highly important U. S. Public Law 91-142 entitled The Education of All Handicapped Children Act of 1975. According to this law:

The term 'children with specific learning disabilities' means those children who have a disorder in one or more of the basic psychological processes involved in understanding or in using language, spoken or written, which disorder may manifest itself in imperfect ability to listen, think, speak, read, write or spell, or do mathematical calculations. Such disorders include such conditions as perceptual handicaps, brain injury, minimal brain dysfunction, dyslexia, and developmental aphasia. Such term does not include children who have learning problems which are primarily the result of visual, hearing, or motor handicaps, of mental retardation, of emotional disturbance, or environmental, cultural, or economic disadvantage (Public Law 94-142, Section 5(b)(4), 1975).

As a follow-up, the U. S. Office of Education (1976) proposed regulations that considered a child to be learning disabled if:

1. The child is not achieving commensurate with his or her age and ability levels in one or more of eight specified areas when provided with learning experiences appropriate for the child's age and ability.
2. There is a severe discrepancy between the child's academic achievement and intellectual ability in one or more of eight specified areas: (1) oral expression, (2) listening comprehension, (3) written expression, (4) basic reading skill, (5) reading comprehension, (6) mathematics calculation, (7) mathematics reasoning, or (8) spelling.

We may note that items (1), (2), (3), and (8) refer to language skills, (4) and (5) specifically to reading, and (6) and (7) to the frequently associated deficiencies in mathematics. However, we should also be mindful that children identified as having learning disabilities are members of a heterogeneous population, as are children who are identified as disabled readers. No child needs to have all of the negative attributes to belong to either group. In fact, whether a child is diagnosed as having a primary reading deficiency or a learning disability often depends upon which clinical specialist first sees him or her. In terms of education and related treatment, each child needs to have his or her problems addressed as they are presented and important to the ultimate objective of teaching the child what he or she needs to learn of language, and of how reading for meaning can be established so that reading becomes a tool for learning. In some instances, reading may also become a way to pleasure. What is appropriate as learning experience must be individualized to the child's best way of learning, rather than to how most children are able to learn.

CHAPTER SEVEN

A Profile of Dyslexia and Dyslexics

What remains true is that the Flauberts were concerned. For a long while Gustave could not grasp the elementary connections that make letters into a syllable, syllables into a word. These difficulties led to others—how can one count without knowing how to read? How can one retain the most basic elements of history and geography if the instruction remains oral? We don't worry about this today; methods are more solid, predictable; and, above all, we take the student *as he is*. At that period there was an order to follow and the child had to bend to it. So Gustave was behind, every step of the way.

His writings hint that . . . the adolescent, like the child before him, never stopped suffering from linguistic malaise or compensating for it by inexpressible ecstasies.

Jean Paul Sartre, *The Family Idiot* (1981)

In my effort to arrive at a profile of the dyslexic child, I reviewed the literature on reading disorders over the past fifty years, with special attention to the publications that included the term *dyslexia* in the title. Despite considerable differences of opinion as to the cause of this severe reading problem, and perhaps even more differences as to how to educate the dyslexic child, the following features were recurrent:

1. Dyslexia occurs more frequently in males than in females. Depending upon the criteria for dyslexia, and the age of the children studied, the male to female ratios ranged from 3 to 1 to 10 to 1. A consensus ratio is from 3 to 4 males for each female. The range estimates change with the age of the children in the studies. The comparative incidence of boys over girls increases with the ages of the children. This suggests that the dyslexic problems are more persistent in boys than in girls and, of course, also in male adults. However, related difficulties in writing may continue to be present in adolescent and adult women.

2. Dyslexics almost always have resistant spelling problems. Letter reversals are prominent, but "bizarre" spellings that do not appear to have any relationship to the spoken word may also be a persistent feature. These deficits may continue to characterize the writing long after proficiency in reading is achieved. Errors in spelling and grammar were present in the writing of such eminent authors as the poet William Butler Yeats and the novelist Agatha Christie.

3. The family background of dyslexics almost always reveals a considerably higher proportion of relatives with reading and learning problems than is found in the population at large.

4. Dyslexia is a constitutional (genetic) disorder. The underlying assumption is that it is an inherited predisposition that is somehow related to atypical organization of the portions of the brain that are involved in the process of learning to read. The unusual brain organization may be a product of maturational delay that initially affects more males than females and is "overcome" earlier in females than in males.

Following is a "tree" of a family that includes three generations and 38 members. Each generation has a considerably higher proportion of reading and learning problems than is found in the population at large, of about 20 percent.

Three Generations of Reading, Writing, and Learning Problems

Grandfather: Reading and learning (R–L) problems

Son No. 1: R–L problems
    four children, two with R–L problems
    12 grandchildren, four with R–L problems

Son No. 2: No R–L problems
    four children, two with R–L problems

Son No. 3: R–L problems
    three children, two with R–L problems
    eight grandchildren, three with R–L problems

Daughter: No R–L problems
    two daughters, one with R–L problems

This family tree was given to me by the grandfather, who identified himself as a dyslexic. He believed, as do I, that the basis for the learning problems was in the underlying early difficulty in learning to read. Of the 38 members in this family "tree," 18 had reading and learning problems. The grandfather and two sons continue to find reading a nonpleasurable task, but they do read with sufficient proficiency to be successful in their vocations and professions. The male-female ratio for R–Ls in this family is 4 to 1.

Kamhi and Catts (1986) compared two groups of children who were identified as having primarily reading disorders or language impairments. On the basis of their investigation, they suggest that these children are not separate populations but may, as individuals, belong to a continuum with related problems. At one end of the continuum are ones whose reading problems are less severe than their language difficulties. At the other end are children with severe reading difficulties but only mild language problems. In any event, reading and learning impairments are often present in the same population.

Following is a two-generation "family tree" that includes five members, all of whom had a history of reading and related early learning problems:

Mother: Reading and learning problems in the first two grades of school. She began to learn to read by a "sounding out" approach in the third grade. She is now an avid reader of materials on all levels of difficulty, professional, technical, fiction and nonfiction, and at least two daily newspapers. Except for maps and spatial directions, she does not think of herself as having any problems associated with dyslexia. Has earned both undergraduate and graduate degrees. She is right-handed.

Father: Had reading difficulty until the middle school grades; was identified as a dyslexic because of poor motor coordination and reading problems. Does not recall any useful instruction in learning how to read, but did somehow teach himself how to solve the written code and was then regarded as a bright student. However, his writing continues to be barely legible, and he is aware of making many errors in spelling. He has advanced degrees in the social sciences, is recognized as preeminent in his field, and is a highly successful writer whose books and articles are cited most frequently by his academic colleagues. He has a distinguished academic career and is now a professor at a prestigious university. He is right-handed, but skillful neither in gross nor in fine coordination.

First son: Had reading problems while in school; spelling poor; handwriting illegible; no difficulty with mathematics. Is said to be ambidextrous but is really ambinondextrous. Has advanced degrees and is a successful writer in his professional field. No problem with reading; was excused from the foreign language requirement for his Ph.D. degree.

Daughter: Reading problems, but less severe than those of her two brothers; improved when transferred from a public to a progressive private school beginning in the fourth grade; can read mirror writing. Has an undergraduate degree from an Ivy League university and a professional master's degree. Is left-handed; has some difficulty in left-right orientation.

Second son: Early reading problems; spelling errors and "minor" grammatical errors; attended an Ivy League university with a major that required considerable reading. Now a successful businessman. Left-handed and has poor gross coordination.

In this family constellation all five members have a history of some degree of reading or learning problems. The intellectual levels and academic achievements of this family are in all instances higher than they are for the population at large and exceptionally high in the light of their early educational problems. Whether the incidence of early problems in the children has a stronger than usual genetic implication is a matter of conjecture. It is also interesting to note that despite the father's high level of academic and professional achievement, he still regards himself as a dyslexic person.

Apparently there is a view among organizations that are concerned with the problems of dyslexia and dyslexic persons that "once a dyslexic, always a dyslexic." The father in the family tree cited above is a recipient of the Margaret Byrd Rawson Society Achievement Award for outstanding accomplishment by a dyslexic adult. In an interview with his university press he said, "After learning how to read, I progessed like a house on fire." As indicated above, he does not do quite as well in spelling. In deference to his secretary and to his own need to read his notes, he often prints his letters instead of writing them.

WHY MORE JOHNNIES THAN JOANNIES?

It is clear from the professional literature that reading problems in males, and especially dyslexic difficulties, have a familial (genetic) basis. However, the specific genetic mechanisms have not yet been determined. Observations about male-female differences, other than dyslexia, should provide a basis for informed speculation.

Up until approximately age 10, girls excel boys in most verbal skills. "Girls are likely to learn to speak earlier, and fewer girls than boys require special remedial instruction in learning to read" (Maccoby, 1966, p. 26). Learning deficits in general are also found in greater proportion among boys than girls. Gates (1961, p. 432), cited in Maccoby and Jacklin (1974, p. 119), concluded that "a relatively large proportion of boys obtained the lowest scores, without a corresponding increase in the number obtaining top scores." In the lower grades, boys outnumbered girls among the lowest scorers by a ratio of 2 to 1.

At the age of 6, when formal reading instruction is begun in the United States, boys are more likely than girls to show the consequences of cerebral lag. Nonreadiness for reading is one of the most serious effects. Psychological results may include frustration, anticipation of failure in all learning activities, and being judged stupid.

Male infants are more likely than females to suffer brain damage at birth as well as prenatal damage. In cases of obvious cerebral palsy, boys outnumber girls by a ratio of about 2 to 1. The same ratio holds for children with so-called minimal brain dysfunction (the M.B.D. syndrome).

Possible Brain Differences

Geschwind and Behan speculated that gender differences might well reflect differences in brain function. Differences in brain function that are related to dyslexia might be a consequence of early exposure to an excess of sex hormones such as testosterone. They note that the male fetus secretes testosterone while in the uterus and so develops a "masculine brain."

Some characteristics of the masculine brain include about a 10 percent greater weight than female brains at maturity and probably a more specialized differentiation between the left and right cerebral hemispheres in regard to language functions. In regard to sex hormones, Hier, a neurologist, supports Geschwind's speculation that "sex hormones may eventually be shown to have important regulatory effects on neural growth, neural regeneration, . . . and neural circuitry" (Hier, 1981, p. 28).

Differences in Language Proficiency and Related Disorders

In this section we will review what we surely know about male-female differences in spoken and written language and other functional differences that I believe have implications for our understanding of dyslexia. Boy babies are a month or two behind girls in beginning to speak.

(There are, of course, numerous exceptions in both directions in regard to language skills as well as other skills to which I will refer. The terms *boys* and *girls* are generalizations.) Girls maintain their advantage over boys at least into the mid-secondary grades in regard to vocabulary size, spelling, grammatical proficiency, and reading. But boys are not without some advantage over girls in some of their own proficiencies such as mathematics, spatial ability, and mechanical skills.

It is, of course, possible that some of the cited differences in skills are a result of cultural influences that maintain initial small advantages. Expectations that begin in early childhood may be expressed in toys and games that we give to and play with children. Thus we may continue what might be minimized if we had no preconceived ideas as to what is appropriate. This, however, is not the position of most developmental psychologists who have observed that boys are likely to learn by doing and acting out and girls—at least most girls—are able to learn in more passive ways. In keeping with this position, it is important to recognize that from kindergarten through the primary grades, women are the teachers, so girls have female models, while boys may have to wait for male models at least until age 10. To generalize, despite early differences, boys are taught how to learn and what to learn by approaches that are usually successful with girls, but in an appreciable number of instances, less successful with boys.

In regard to difficulties and disorders of spoken and written language, boys consistently outnumber girls. Considerably more boys than girls have serious language delay, both in comprehension and production of speech. Boys have more problems in articulation and in the production of cluttered speech and stuttering. It is of interest to note that the ratio for stuttering is 4 males to 1 female, as it is for dyslexia. Geschwind noted that boys outnumber girls in the special populations of the hyperactive and those who are identified as having behavior problems while in school.

Implications of the Observed Sex Ratio Differences

If we accept the still speculative neurophysiological and neuropsychological explanations of the causes of the established male-female differences, what are the implications for when and how we should teach children to read? A pessimistic implication is that we will continue to have many more males than females with reading problems, some so severe as to be designated as dyslexic. A less pessimistic observation is that we may be able to teach male children, and a much smaller proportion of female children, to learn to read by teaching them differently from most of their peer-age children. These differences should include using approaches that are compatible with their learning styles and cognitive abilities and beginning to teach reading at a later age, perhaps as late as 8 or even 9 in some instances, allowing time for the children's neurological system to mature. In his summary of a recent Conference on Sex Differences in Dyslexia, Masland (1981) states: "To be successful, instruction must be appropriate to the individual regardless of sex." Masland also notes: "Above all, the conference continually highlighted that the differences among individuals are far more significant than are the differences between sexes." As a general observation, the approach to the dyslexic child, regardless of sex or age, should be to "exploit his (her) natural strategy rather than attempt to correct or strengthen his (her) area of deficit." How this can be done will be considered later.

For the present we should be mindful that dyslexia is not a unitary disorder but a complex of overlapping syndromes. Some of these were considered in Chapter Six. Nevertheless, a fundamental question to consider is whether boys, because they do have better spatial skills than girls, should have initial instruction in reading through a whole-word approach. However, it is also possible that girls who are dyslexic resemble boys in their neuro-organizational systems and thus would also benefit from a whole-word approach in early stages of remediation. This recommendation does not argue against so-called phonetic teaching for both boys and girls in later stages of reading instruction. I do think it important for children who have adequate hearing to become aware that however inconsistently in English, the alphabet does have some relationship to how a word is represented in writing.

In the final analysis, each child should be observed and assessed so that the teacher can become aware of the child's cognitive style, how she or he best learns what the school has to teach. If a child fails to learn by a given method or approach, persistent use of the method may be destructive. If reading must be taught because the child is in a given grade at a given chronological age, the use of an alternative method that does no violence to his or her cognitive style for other forms of learning is a minimal requisite.

ERRORS AND INACCURACIES OF IMPROFICIENT READERS AND DYSLEXICS

Children who are in the early stages of learning to read and to write are likely to reverse letters such as *d* and *b* and *p* and *q* and make upside-down reversal in writing such as *w* for *m*. They are also prone to making letter order reversals such as *pats* for *past*, *was* for *saw*, and *on* for *no*.

Left   Hand   Right

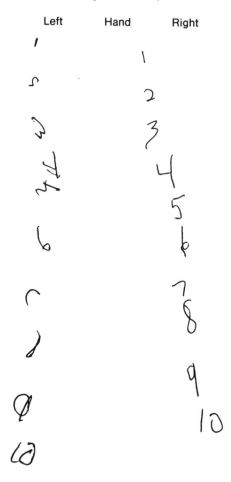

FIGURE 7–1. Example of writing of digits of a left-handed adult with a history of reading problems. Subject was changed to write with the right hand in early school grades, but except for writing, remains left-handed. Instructions for the sample were, "Close your eyes and write quickly, both hands at once, a column of digits from 1 to 10."

Letter order reversals may also produce such results as *gib* for *big*, and *teps* for *pets*. Errors such as these are corrected by children who read for meaning and become aware of letter order reversals that produce nonsense sequences. A few children somehow manage to reverse the entire sequence of letters and do mirror-writing as well as mirror-reading. Other early errors include omissions of letters and of words in writing

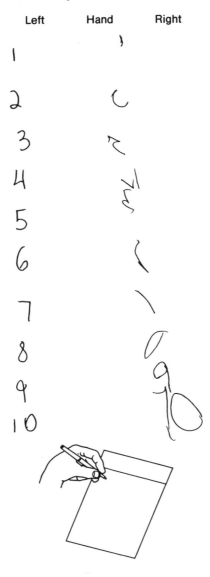

FIGURE 7–2. Sample of writing of digits (eyes closed) by a left-handed adult with no history of reading or writing problems. Note that the reversals were made by the right hand. The drawing indicates the hand position for usual cursive writing for this adult.

and reading and substitution of words. When word substitutions do not alter the meaning of the material in context, I regard them as an indicator that the child is reading for meaning and, therefore, as a good prognosticator of future reading ability. Common errors in writing of numbers are ⊬ for 4 and Г for 7.

These errors usually are corrected as the children grow older. They seldom occur, except in situations of stress, by the time the child is in the third grade. When children are writing rapidly, these errors may appear again. The most frequent errors made in typing (typos) are letter reversals, letter order sequencing, and omissions of words. Improficient readers, expecially dyslexics, continue to make errors that are characteristic of the productions of young children. The persistence of these errors is an expression of the disability and not the underlying cause or causes of reading problems.

Frequent eye-movement errors of disabled readers include left-right confusion, short and erratic eye sweeps, and long pauses between eye sweeps. These eye (oculomotor) movements are known to be related to proficiency in reading. The meaning of what the eyes see is "established" at the moment of pause between sweeps. Research evidence indicates that the faulty eye movements are the result rather than the causes of reading problems. There is no evidence to support the assumption that the practice of subjecting a dyslexic to oculomotor training will, of itself, improve reading comprehension. Research on eye-movement errors, including his own studies, is reviewed by Rayner (1983). Rayner reports that when two adult dyslexics were given material to read on the level of their tested reading ability, about the third grade to fourth grade, their eye-movement patterns were similar to those of third- and fourth-graders. However, when the subjects were given more difficult material, their eye-movement patterns became irregular.

Changes in eye-movement patterns such as regressions, reversals, and increased time between sweeps are probably characteristic of all of us who are reading difficult material. Those of us who have only partial ability with a second language are likely to have short eye sweeps and reread to make certain that we do, in fact, understand what we are trying to read.

MOTOR TRAINING FOR DYSLEXICS

In the 1950s and 1960s, clinics and other agencies that had dyslexic children as clients were providing training in such activities as trampoline jumping, narrow rail walking, and crawling through elongated barrels. The assumption presumably was that because of a fair number of children with reading problems had left-right confusion and perhaps a lack of awareness of their bodies in space, such training would establish appropriate brain-hemisphere dominance and therefore, somehow, dominance and control for reading. There is no scientific research evidence to support either the assumption or the conclusion that such practices make for more efficient reading. It is possible, if the training covers a long enough period and the child succeeds in these gymnastic exercises, that he or she will feel more accomplished than before the training began. Further, growing a year or two older while the formal teaching of reading is postponed may allow for sufficient neurophysiologic maturity to make reading readiness possible. Pirozzolo (1979, p. 87) presents this view of relevant research and irrelevant practices as follows:

Neuropsychological research has provided some very valuable scientific information about "why Johnny can't read." The name of science has been tarnished by pseudoscientists who claim that they can decrease the incidence of dyslexia by using a specific reading program, or teach a child to read by training him to crawl, or remediate any reading difficulty by using special instrumentation. The challenge for future research on the neuropsychology of developmental reading disorders is to determine the exact functional losses in reading disability and find some appropriate methods for working with individual children. Experience in the rehabilitation of brain-damaged patients has clearly shown that the most important factor is not the method but the patient's relationship with the therapist. The recognition that it is the psychological contact between teacher and student that is the basis for learning rather than the program or method is the most important practical message that neuropsychology has communicated.

Although I do not minimize importance of the choice of approach or method in the teaching of reading to disabled readers, I am in total agreement as to the importance of the relationship in the teaching of *reading at any time.* Moreover, there are dysfunctioning methods and there are dysfunctioning teachers, the latter, perhaps, because they are burdened with a prescribed method for all children, who are expected to learn to read because they have "become of age."

CHAPTER EIGHT

The Dyslexic in School and Society

I could not reed
I could not rite
But I could steal
And I could fite.

Dyslexic School Dropout
(Adolescent Delinquent)

In this chapter we shall review the progress, the fortunes—and all too often the misfortunes—of dyslexics beyond the elementary school years. We shall find a disportionately high number of delinquents among them who are school failures despite average to superior intelligence. We shall also find some dyslexics who persevere and succeed in higher education and in the professions as well as in the arts and literature. We shall also present an "Honor Roll" of dyslexics who, by the most stringent standards, are persons of eminence.

DYSLEXIA AND DELINQUENCY

It is clear from a variety of studies that there is an unfortunate but positive relationship between dyslexia and delinquency. However, it is not clear whether delinquents are prone to become dyslexic or whether the socially undesirable behaviors are the responses to the problems of reading and writing difficulties that make early and later efforts in school frustrating experiences. It may well be that those who fail and drop out of school and later become identified delinquents do so because of other environmental or innate factors, or a combination of both, that make delinquency a way out of immediate frustration. My own review of the literature does little to cut or unravel the "Gordian knot" of this relationship.

Mulligan (1969) found severe reading disability in 39 of 49 adolescents whose delinquencies were serious enough to make them eligible for commitment to the California Youth Authority. Mulligan notes that:

"Typically, these delinquent children are of average to superior intelligence, but because of their handicap they are unable to achieve in the regular school setting. . . . Their school problems begin when they reach the level where they are supposed to learn to read.

On the basis of her own study and a survey of the literature, Andrew (1981) found poor reading ability to be common to most delinquents. She suggests that "Reading may . . . emerge as a marker variable rather than as a primary cause of delinquency."

Observations along the same lines are made by Thomson (1984), a British psychologist, educator, and writer and the Principal of the East Court School for Dyslexic Children in London. Thomson generalizes that:

The acquisition of written language can be a very stressful process for many children; many pressures from both home and school are focussed on the child to make him succeed. The dyslexics' difficulties will include the unhappy anxious boy of eight, misperceived by teachers; the behavioural disorders of 12 and 13-year-olds referred to the school psychological services for treatment; the so called "disabled illiterate school leaver" described by the Department of Employment; the frustrated science, engineering or medical students unable to present their very able thinking in written form; the referrals to psychiatric hospitals of men in the 30–40 age range whose breakdowns are traced back to inabilities to read and write; and the high incidence of illiteracy amongst young offenders in penal establishments. (Thomson, 1984, p. 20)

Thomson's sweeping observations emphasize the problems and misfortunes of dyslexics. But many dyslexics do learn to deal with their problems, some so successfully that they should no longer be considered dyslexic. Nevertheless, reading and writing difficulties may continue into and beyond the secondary school grades and constitute a challenge to learning. Fortunately, some dyslexics receive help for their improficiencies in reading and writing in selected educational institutions. The best of these institutions (special schools) are aware that despite the common term *dyslexia*, as individuals, no two dyslexics are alike. Specific symptoms and degree of difficulty vary considerably one from the other. Fortunately, so do their strengths. Remediation, to be successful, must take both the weaknesses and the strengths of a student into consideration in an individually devised or adapted custom-made program, which should be arrived at by rational choice and psychological insight rather than by chance.

In the next chapter we shall review several specialized approaches that are in current use with children and adolescents identified as dyslexics. For the present we will consider adjustments that are made by some secondary schools and colleges for dyslexic students.

SECONDARY SCHOOLS

Remedial instruction for dyslexic students in the secondary schools ranges widely in approach and objectives. Some schools, more often those that are private and require tuition fees comparable to those of Ivy League colleges, offer individualized programs that include in-depth diagnosis, counseling, and instruction in reading and writing, as well as the academic course work for college admission. The best of public schools may do as well if there is parent interest and adequate funding. At worst, in some public schools, dyslexic students, among others in attendance, are promoted on an age rather than achievement basis and eventually are "graduated" from high school as functional illiterates. In still other school districts, dyslexic students are assigned to vocational training, presumably on the assumption that only a minimum amount of ability to read and write is required.

In the best academic situations, whether in public or private schools, psychodiagnosis, psychological counseling, and remedial instruction in reading are available. Psychodiagnosis is intended to determine personality problems that may be the reaction to the dyslexic involvements or, in some instances, aggravate and maintain these problems as a fall-back explanation for low achievement. Psychodiagnosis also helps to determine a student's profile of potential strengths and present weaknesses to provide a basis for the remedial instruction. Essential information includes the most effective intake modality—visual, auditory, or in some instances, moto-kinesthetic. Such information should influence, if not dictate, how to individualize a teaching program.

Other academic adjustments include balancing a student's schedule so that nonreading or "light" reading courses are taken along with one or two that require "heavy" reading. Most programs encourage students with reading difficulties to enroll in fewer courses than are usually carried during a school quarter or semester, at least until the student feels secure enough in reading proficiency and writing to carry a full schedule. In some instances such scheduling may require an added year of school or attendance during one or two summer sessions to complete the academic requirements for graduation.

TREATMENT PROGRAMS

Despite recent evidence that dyslexic persons do not conform to a single pattern of basic or related dysfunctions, in practice, treatment programs are not as individualized as we might expect. In 1976, in his book *Investigating the Issues of Reading Disabilities*, Spache observed,

"Surprisingly, despite the great variety of signs and symptoms that are assumed to characterize dyslexia, recommended treatments are few in number" (p. 185). Although the situation is somewhat improved today, remedial instructional programs that may begin in the elementary grades and continue into the secondary schools are likely to be one of the following:

1. Multisensory stimulation, usually combining two or more sensory avenues (visual-auditory-kinesthetic- or tactile impressions). These, in selected combination, may be provided simultaneously or in quick succession.

2. Training in perceptual-motor and eye-hand coordination.

3. Phonics, often combined with one of the above.

4. Training in nonverbal and verbal situations to overome weaknesses in auditory or visual perception and sequencing of events.

5. Language "enrichment" to establish an increased functional vocabulary, awareness of grammatical structures, and correction of spelling.

6. Reading skills that emphasize meaning in context rather than so-called phonetic "decoding." Depth of comprehension rather than speed of reading is stressed.

Advocates of multisensory programs such as the Gillingham-Stillman and other variations of the initial Orton-Gillingham approach are showing an increasing awareness of the need to enhance the linguistic knowledge of dyslexics. Accordingly, their programs include establishing knowledge of sentence structure, vocabulary building, and language comprehension. For example, Cox (1985) describes a program that specifically includes the teaching of syntax, verbal expression, semantics, thought, and imagination. An important addition is listening to selected "good" literature to improve comprehension skills and to provide an appreciation of our literary heritage.

PROGRESS OF SECONDARY SCHOOL STUDENTS IN PROGRAMS FOR DYSLEXICS

Earlier we considered the high incidence of delinquency and emotional problems in the dyslexic population. Fortunately, there is also a bright side to the picture. Most dyslexics, as children and adults, do cope with their problems, and most overcome them. Many dyslexics, especially those who are identified early and are of average or above-average intelligence, and are fortunate in receiving appropriate education, do well in schools and in their vocations and professions. A long-term follow-up study by three Johns Hopkins University investigators is particularly encouraging. Finucci, Gottfredson, and Childs (1985) reported on more than 500 men who had attended an independent private school for boys, and all of whom had been identified as having developmental dyslexia. The study covered a period of from 1 to 38 years after the students had left their school. The investigators found that:

1. More than half the number had graduated from college.
2. While at college, most of the students majored in business.
3. After leaving college, most were employed in managerial or related business positions.
4. On what we might consider the negative side, as adults their reading interests and habits did not compare favorably with those of other men of similar socioeconomic background without a history of dyslexia, with whom the subjects of the study were compared.

Is this report typical of results obtained in other schools and programs for dyslexic students? Frankly, I do not know. It is likely that successes are more frequently reported than are failures. Nor do we know how many of the students enrolled in special schools might have overcome their dyslexic difficulties on their own. We do know from many anecdotal reports that despite improvement in reading, persons with a history of dyslexia admit to being poor spellers and not a few to finding grammar a continuing mystery.

Eileen Simpson, a clinical psychologist and author, cites the errors in spelling and grammar of several well-known authors, as well as her continued difficulties in spelling and slow reading. Her autobiographical book, *Reversals: A Personal Account of Victory Over Dyslexia* (1979) notes such errors as *olny* for *only, deare* for *dear, gary* for *gray* (reversals), and *swimmiming* for *swimming*. These errors were made in a letter that contained 25 words. Simpson believes that she has now won her victory over dyslexia, not because she is symptom free, but because her symptoms are manageable "at least on good days" (p. 217).

HIGHER EDUCATION

Colleges and professional schools provide new challenges for students with a history of dyslexia. Even those students whose hard-earned proficiencies in reading and writing were adequate in secondary schools may be faced with new and more difficult expectations in higher and professional education. Demands for reading, for writing reports and term papers, which are especially heavy in liberal arts programs, and the need to write final examinations under pressure may constitute conditions "hazardous to student well being."

Until fairly recently, many students with a history of dyslexia who managed to get through college did so by wit, grit, and sometimes deception. "Adjustments" to demands take many forms. With the instructor's approval, recitations and lectures may be recorded and played back at leisure. Friendly classmates may make copies of their notes for students who cannot readily listen and write their own notes. Some fraternities and, I assume, some sororities provide class notes to their members and may, usually legitimately, keep a file of past examinations in selected courses. Less scrupulous students—a lack of scruples is not peculiar to dyslexics—may engage other students to write their reports and term papers.

Fortunately, the situation is changing. Though wit and grit are still positive attributes, deception is no longer necessary. Most colleges are now making adjustments for dyslexic students. Though dyslexics may have to work harder than their peers and possibly take a year longer to complete the requirements for their degrees, they do not find the academic doors closed to them. Brown University is one of the Ivy League schools that provides support services for dyslexic students. Each student is treated on an ad hoc basis. A student may exercise an option to take a reduced course load and complete graduation requirements in five years with each year's tuition pro-rated. By pre-arrangement, additional time may be given for examinations. In some instances, oral examinations are permitted. Individual tutoring is available to teach dyslexic students how to structure sentences and organize sentences into coherent paragraphs. The use of word-processors and typewriters that alert the writer to spelling errors helps considerably in reducing the frustration and time pressures of ordinary typewriting.

Brown University's interest in dyslexic students is explained by Katherine Hinds (1985). In an interview with Dean Robert Shaw of the College, the interviewer was impressed that in addition to a sincere desire to help the students, there is the "perception that the federal government requires us to help them in the same way as the law requiring that Brown have handicap access for students in wheelchairs." Brown is considered in the forefront in providing services for these students.

Although many colleges now make adjustments for dyslexic students, Landmark College in Vermont was organized exclusively for precollege and college students with dyslexic and related learning problems. Landmark provides instruction that emphasizes both oral and written language skills, for the most part on a one-to-one tutorial basis. Landmark opened its doors for dyslexic students in September, 1985. Landmark also operates elementary and secondary schools for children with learning problems in Massachusetts and California (Meyer, 1986).

DYSLEXIA IN PERSONS OF EMINENCE

This chapter opened with a discussion of dyslexia and delinquency. It will close with a selected list—an Honor Roll—of eminent persons who had an early history of dyslexic difficulties. (The sources for this selection include Thompson, 1979; Critchley & Critchley, 1978; and my own biographical research.)

An Annotated Selected List of Eminent Persons Who Were Dyslexic

Hans Christian Andersen (1805–1875): Danish novelist, poet, and writer of fairy tales; recognized as Denmark's foremost author and story-teller.

Niels Bohr (1885–1962): Danish physicist; much of contemporary thinking in physics is based on Bohr's theories of the structure of the atom; awarded the Nobel Prize in Physics in 1922.

Dame Agatha Christie (1891–1977): British novelist most famous for her detective stories; the author of more than 80 books; also published novels under the pseudonym of Mary Westmacott.

Dr. Harvey Cushing (1869–1939): American neurosurgeon, teacher, and biographer; in 1925 was awarded the Pulitzer Prize for his biography of Sir William Osler, a famous Canadian physician and medical historian.

Leonardo da Vinci (1452–1519): Italian Renaissance genius; artist, architect, sculptor, musician, engineer, and scientist.

Thomas Alva Edison (1847–1931): American inventor whose special genius was in the practical application of scientific principles. His inventions include the phonograph, the first practical incandescent (carbon filament) light bulb, electrical distribution systems, and electric generators. The name Edison is included in many regional electric utility systems in the United States. Was essentially self-taught beyond the basic teaching by his mother; had about three months of primary school teaching in a school in Port Huron, Michigan; was withdrawn from school because he was considered a "backward" child not capable of learning. An early illness (scarlet fever) resulted in later hearing impairment.

George Patton, Jr. (1885–1945): United States general during World War II; commanded the Third Army, which was responsible for successful operations in France and Germany. Patton was a "weak" and unhappy student while at West Point. He had considerable difficulty in reading but had an excellent memory for what he heard and managed to read. This special ability enabled him to memorize and reproduce entire lectures and texts.

Nelson A. Rockefeller (1908–1979): American public official and philanthropist; Vice-President of the United States and three times governor of New York State; did considerable writing on issues of governmental reorganization and preservation of the environment.

Auguste Rodin (1840–1917): French artist and sculptor; most famous sculptures are *The Thinker, The Burghers of Calais,* and his monuments to Honoré de Balzac and Victor Hugo. As a child he did poorly in all school subjects, presumably because he was near-sighted.

Thomas Woodrow Wilson (1856–1924): After serving as president of Princeton University and as Governor of New Jersey, was elected as the twenty-eighth President of the United States. Wilson wrote the Covenant for the League of Nations. His numerous writings include essays and books on jurisprudence and political science.

William Butler Yeats (1865–1939): Irish poet and playwright; a major figure of twentieth-century literature; recognized as the leader of the Irish literary renaissance. Founded the Irish Literary Theater in Dublin; awarded the Nobel Prize in Literature in 1923. Yeats is considered Ireland's most famous lyric poet.

Albert Einstein (1879–1955): It is not clear whether Albert Einstein was dyslexic as a child or so different in his thinking and his responses to formal education that biographers have difficulty in explaining his early undistinguished academic history. Einstein was born in Germany and lived in Switzerland and Italy. His early work history as an examiner for the patent office in Bern, Switzerland did not suggest his future greatness as a physicist. Nevertheless, he earned his doctor's degree and evolved his theory of relativity during this period of employment—from 1902 to 1909—as an examiner. Perhaps the low intellectual demands of his employment allowed him the time he needed for the thinking and theoretic formulations for which he became famous. Einstein was awarded the Nobel Prize in Physics in 1921. He became a citizen of the United States in 1940.

Ronald Clark, one of Einstein's biographers (1971), states that:

Nothing in Einstein's early history suggests dormant genius. Quite the contrary. The one feature of his childhood about which there appears no doubt is the lateness with which he learned to speak. Even at the age of nine he was not fluent, while reminiscences of his youth stress hesitancies and the fact that he would reply to questions only after consideration and reflection. His parents feared that he might be subnormal, and it has even been suggested that in his infancy he may have suffered from a form of dyslexia. (pp. 9–10)

There may be come confusion as to the definition of the syndrome of dyslexia. Delay in onset of speech and early hesitancies are not, in themselves, indicative of dyslexia, and it is not a disability of infancy but of childhood when reading and writing difficulties become apparent. In regard to delay of onset of speaking, I prefer to believe that young Albert was waiting to find someone who could understand what he had to say before bothering to talk.

Other Dyslexics

Names of other eminent persons are included in publications about dyslexics or others with early learning and language problems. Thompson (1971) includes Paul Ehrlich (German bacteriologist), William James (American psychologist), Abbott Lawrence Lowell (President of Harvard University, 1909–1931), and his sister, Amy Lowell (poet and literary critic).

Gustave Flaubert (1821–1880) is another name cited by biographers of dyslexics (e.g., Simpson, 1979, and Sartre, 1981). Flaubert is regarded by critics as among the most eminent of French novelists, and particularly as a master of the realistic novel. He wrote slowly and with scrupulous care that each word would be the exact word (*le mot juste*). His masterpiece and probably his best known novel, *Madame Bovary*, was five years in the writing. Was Flaubert dyslexic? Did he have learning disabilities as a child? Did he develop so slowly and so differently that his family considered him to be at best retarded and at worst, the family idiot?

Paul Sartre, whose biography of Gustave Flaubert is called *The Family Idiot* (1981), provides his explanation to "set the record straight." According to Sartre, Gustave was an ailing child whose mother cared for him physically but found it difficult to love him or to understand him. Gustave is described as ". . . a simple soul, improbably, pathologically credulous; he frequently fell into long stupors—his parents searched his features and feared he was an idiot." Sartre presents his view of the mother's lack of sympathy and understanding of Gustave's behavior and development as a child and even as an adult when he had achieved recognition for his writing.

> . . . she never believed in her son's genius or even in his talent. In the first place, these words had no meaning for her; as the widow of a brain, brains alone were worthy of her respect. As a practical person, she recognized talent only in *capable* men who were valued as such, since their capability allowed them to sell their services for a higher price. (p. 7)

Gustave Flaubert's father was an affluent surgeon. Presumably, the mother could respect only persons whose brains could be put to proper use. Gustave did not fall into this practical category.

Sartre does recognize that as an adolescent, Gustave's spelling was "somewhat fanciful" and that the child did not learn to read until age 7 or 8. This may have been late for members of his family. However, as a child, Gustave enjoyed listening to stories and was fortunate that he had adults to read to him. It is also likely that because he was a sickly child, he had the benefit of more listening to reading than most other children. In any event, despite his spelling, he surely caught up!

DYSLEXIA AS A CHALLENGE

It is obvious from our selected list of persons of eminence who had a history of developmental dyslexia and related language and learning problems that the difficulties and their frequent consequences can be overcome. Some were men and women who throughout their lives could not quite master the mystery of spelling. Others had to be continuously vigilant about correct grammar, but despite or possibly because of these improficiencies, were able in time to achieve eminence. In impressive incidence, extraordinary levels of achievement were reached in literature. A simplistic explanation is that literary achievement in persons who were once severely dyslexic represents over-compensation. Without doubt, our culture is enriched by this drive.

Many dyslexics make vocational adjustments and choose fields of employment that do not demand much reading or writing. Others go into professions such as law and medicine that make heavy demands for reading and writing but adjust to these demands by extra time and effort. Several of my colleagues who must "publish or perish" in the academic world still regard themselves as dyslexics. Among them are scholars with notable and deserved reputations for their scholarship and writings. For all such persons, the most eminent and the near-eminent, for the teachers and the writers, dyslexia did not become an excuse for failure.

What characterizes those who succeed despite their early and sometimes persistent background of language and learning difficulties and those who find these difficulties unsurmountable obstacles? Why is there so much delinquency in striking contrast to the evidence of eminence? The highest level of intellectual genius may be one factor, but there may well be other influences, innate or environmental, or a combination of both, that contribute, at least in part, to the difference in achievement. If for no other reason than the importance of the contributions to our society made by dyslexic persons of eminence, and those on a lesser level who make their own contributions, we must make a determined effort to learn the answers.

CHAPTER NINE

Nondyslexic Children at High Risk for Reading Failure

> If it were not for the capacity for ambiguity, for the sensing of
> strangeness, that words in all languages provide, we would
> have no way of recognizing the layers of counterpoint in mean-
> ing, and we might be spending all our time sitting on stone
> fences, staring into the sun. . . . The great thing about
> human language is that it prevents us from sticking to the
> matter at hand.
>
> Lewis Thomas, *The Lives of a Cell* (1975)

A sizable population of school-age children are at high risk for failure to
learn to read but are not primarily dyslexic. These populations include
children with severe disorders of articulation (the dysarthric and dyspraxic), those who are severely delayed in their onset and development
of spoken language (the aphasic), and those with severe hearing impairments (the deaf). We may add to these special groups, all of whom have a
physical (organic) underlying cause for their high-risk status, the ever
increasing number of children for whom English is a second language
and who may not have adequate exposure to speakers of English, or who
have not been motivated to learn to speak English before they enter the
primary school grades.

CHILDREN WITH SEVERE DISORDERS OF ARTICULATION

Not included in this high-risk population are children with so-called
infantile speech. In their early career as speakers these children lisp or
substitute a *w* quality sound for *l* or *r* or omit or transpose sounds and
often syllables within words, as in *nubby* for *bunny*. Most of these
"garden variety" of articulation and pronunciation errors are corrected
by the time the child enters the elementary school grades. By age 7, at
least 75 percent of children, girls about a month to 6 months ahead of

boys, are in control of the speech sounds of their language. In some instances, full control is not achieved until age 8 or 9. About 2 percent of children may continue to lisp, and some to have other habitual errors in articulation. Children with a variety of speech errors are also likely to be those with an over-all language proficiency problem and so be at some risk for reading difficulty. I am not including in this group children with organic problems such as cleft palate, cerebral palsy, or hearing impairment.

Unless there is an organic basis for articulation problems, "garden variety" misarticulations do not interfere with normal language learning and so with learning to read. However, severe articulation disorders that have a neurological cause have more serious implications for learning to read, especially when there is evidence of brain damage and even more so when the child is retarded in understanding spoken language. These children are identified as *dysarthric* and *dyspraxic*.

Dysarthria

Dysarthria is the technical term for articulation disorders that result from nervous system damage. Severe articulation deficits that make it difficult even for members of the family to understand what the child is trying to say are often accompanied by initial language delay and later by over-all language improficiency characterized by a sparse vocabulary and slow acquisition of the grammar of the language.

Dysarthric children are likely to distort or to omit sounds that are difficult for them, such as *r, l, s, z, t, d, p,* and *b.* They may omit entire syllables that include difficult sounds. In severe cases, such as in children with cerebral palsy, the entire speech effort is so disordered as to be unintelligible except possibly to those family members who are closest to them.

Such children are not likely to be ready for reading at the usual age at which formal teaching is undertaken in most public schools in the United States and Great Britain, that is, about age 6. If reading is taught by an approach that depends on oral (spoken) initial "decoding"—the so-called phonic method—the child is certainly at a high risk for early failure and for being turned away from trying to learn to read when, at a later age and with more knowledge of language, he or she may be ready to deal with written language.

If the pressures, either from the family or from the school system, are such that despite negative indicators—dysarthric difficulties and language improficiency—reading is to be directly taught, the approach should bypass the need for articulating and a visual-to-visual approach be employed. This approach should provide a basic working vocabulary and grammatical constructions in an order that is consistent with the acquisitions of normal hearing children. *Reading for Meaning* (Eisenson, 1984b) is such a program. This and other visual programs will be considered later.

Oral Dyspraxia

Dyspraxia means a disability to perform coordinated movements for an intended propose. Oral (articulatory) dyspraxia is a disorder in the voluntary control of the muscles involved in speech production. Literally, the organs of articulation do not execute the speaker's bidding. As a consequence, the sounds of speech may be distorted or out of sequence, or both. In some instances, articulation resembles a young child's production so that *banana* is produced as *naba* (sounds transposed and others omitted) and *doggy* may come out as *goddy*. A longer word such as *spaghetti* may have variable productions such as *pasghetti*, and *gaspetti* and *gappi*. The last reflects the dyspraxic child's tendency to omit sounds and entire syllables, possibly in an effort to simplify articulation. Dyspraxia is characterized by inconsistency of production. Another feature, much like the efforts of children who are just beginning to speak, is to omit the first sound of a sound blend. Blends of consonant sounds occur frequently in English as *sp* (spoon, spot); *st* (stand, stew, best); *pl* (play, please, apple); *bl* (blue, blow); *br* (bring, bread); *fr* (frame, friend); *gr* (grow, ground); *nd* (and, stand, friend, ground). A particularly difficult blend is the *sk* (sky, skin, ask). Even more difficult are the triple consonant blends, as in *asks*, *pests*, *spring*, *fists*, and *wants* and *stray*. These "tongue twisters" defy many young children and even some adults who continue to pronounce *asks* as *aks* or as the easier production, *asts*.

An early indicator of possible oral dyspraxia is persistent drooling, difficulty in chewing food, and gagging. In some instances, oral dyspraxia is accompanied by a general awkwardness and incoordination of movements. Fortunately, most children improve as they mature. A few do not.

It is evident that because a dyspraxic child has an untrustworthy articulation mechanism, in teaching him or her to read, we must bypass the need to articulate. Accordingly, the phonic approach is not an acceptable choice. However, unless they are "turned off" as speakers and cease to listen because they are not understood in their turn, dysarthric and dyspraxic children should be encouraged to listen even though they cannot engage in easy two-way communications. Unless the child is also significantly delayed in spoken language comprehension, reading may be taught to the school-age child by a visual-to-visual approach. We will present such approaches after our consideration of the congenitally deaf. First, however, we will consider a fascinating population of brain-different children—the aphasic and dysphasic—who have listening rather than hearing problems and are all too often confused with the deaf.

APHASIA AND DYSPHASIA

Another group of children who are at high risk for reading failure are the aphasic and dysphasic, unless they are taught by alternatives to the "usual" methods of teaching.

Literally, dysphasia implies a lesser degree of severity than aphasia. However, the practice in Great Britain and in European countries is to use the term *dysphasia* with modifying words such as *mild, moderate,* or *severe* to indicate degrees of impairment.

Congenitally aphasic children are the most seriously delayed in language development who are not also mentally retarded, deaf, or autistic (nonrelating, emotionally disturbed). These children are *brain different* either because of delay in the maturation of the areas of the brain that process (receive and decode) spoken language or because of actual damage to the brain before birth, during the birth process, or shortly after birth. Because congenitally aphasic children cannot decode spoken language within the age range of normal children, they are also severely impaired in learning to speak. They do, however, understand nonspeech sounds such as animal noises, and in general, the mechanical noises of their environment. Their inability to understand spoken language and to make themselves understood often results in confusion and misdiagnosis so that they may be considered "peculiarly" deaf because they do respond appropriately to nonspeech sounds, or mentally retarded, or emotionally disturbed.

Early acquired aphasia is appropriately used for children who learned to speak normally and then, because of illness of accident, suffered damage to the brain with consequent impairment in their ability to understand or produce speech. If the child's brain damage is limited to one hemisphere of the brain, the likelihood is that he or she will rather quickly recover from most of the impairments for spoken language. However, there is also a likelihood that the child will have difficulty with reading if he or she had learned to read, or more difficulty in learning to read as a new experience.

HEARING AND LISTENING

Hearing and listening need to be distinguished for several reasons that are related to the understanding of speech. Some aphasic children do, in fact, have mild hearing losses, about the equivalent of the reduced hearing when we suffer from a common cold. This amount of loss would not in itself impair or significantly delay speech development in a child who is not also brain different. Among aphasic children, however, this amount of loss compounds their difficulty in attempting to understand— to listen and decode—what is said to them. When speech is slowed down, but not at the expense of the speech melody (intonation), and the quantity of the messages is reduced, the aphasic child may be able to comprehend. This is especially so if something visual is associated with the spoken language. Fortunately, most aphasic children have no difficulty in understanding what they see. This may be so because visual events usually are static and do not change in character as we look at them. Unless we are attending to moving pictures, or are ourselves moving quickly past visual situations, we can take a second look or, if we choose, look as long as we please without concern that what we are looking at will change. In contrast, when we are engaged in listening, the events change physically and continuously. We must resort to memory to organize what we just heard—listened to—while we are involved in listening to whatever is occurring at the moment. The moment is, in fact, a small fraction of a second. *Auditory events fade into history while they are being produced.* Aphasic children are impaired in this organizational ability. They are, in effect, slow listeners. This ability improves with maturation, especially if they are identified early in their preschool years and are given specialized instruction. (The identification and treatment of aphasic children is considered in detail in Eisenson, 1984a.)

Unless aphasic children have widespread brain damage that involves both hemispheres, almost all of them who have adequate intelligence do learn language and consequently should be able to learn to read. However, even with specialized instruction, many of them take until age 9 before they learn as much language as an average 4- or 5-year-old child. It follows that the teaching of reading should be delayed unless such teaching also provides basic language instruction that includes opportunity for learning the grammar of the language in ways that parallel normal language acquisition. A second recommendation is to minimize or, at least initially, to bypass spoken language and to teach reading on a visual-to-visual basis so that the printed words have associated specific

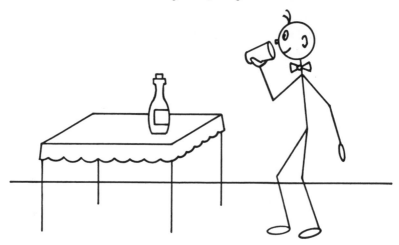

Figure 9–1. "Boy drinks."

visual illustrations to "dictate" the meaning. An example is the illustration for "Boy drinks." Other examples will be provided in the later discussion of Reading for Meaning: An Illustrated Language Acquisition Program.

THE DEAF

One child per 1,000 is born with hearing impairment so severe that they are designated as deaf. Practically, a child may be considered to be deaf if the impairment of hearing is so severe that even with appropriate amplification, vision rather than hearing becomes the main avenue for language learning and communication. In terms of objective measurement of hearing loss, with few exceptions, the use of vision as the primary avenue for communication occurs when the impairment in hearing is about 90 decibels (Quigley & King, 1984, p. 1).

The *deafened* are those who suffer severe loss of hearing after they have learned to speak well enough for speech to become the primary avenue for communication. Unlike the congenitally deaf, these children are not likely to be severely retarded in language proficiency and can learn to read with established language as a basis for this new achievement.

Language Proficiency and Deafness

The vast majority of congenitally deaf children, as well as adolescents and adults, are seriously retarded in language proficiency in general and reading and writing proficiency in particular. This lack of proficiency refers to the use of conventional language that is based on the ability to hear, understand, and produce spoken language. This is obviously not fair to the deaf, whose sign systems enable them to communicate adequately with other persons who share their system. However, though the situation may change with increased use of sign systems that incorporate "conventional" grammatical features, compared with most hearing persons, almost all deaf persons are poor readers.

Following are some observations by authorities on the deaf:

The poverty that deaf children show in their understanding and use of English, especially in the light of their rich linguistic potential as human beings is most distressing. (Kretschmer & Kretschmer, 1978, p. 130)

On the basis of their review of recent literature and their investigations, Quigley and Paul (1984) note:

The median reading score at age 20 years and older was a grade equivalent of 4.5. Only about 10% of students in the best reading group (18 years of age) could read at or above the eighth-grade level.

The reading ability of the deaf in Great Britain is no better than it is in the United States. An illustrative study by Conrad (1977) found that on leaving school at 15 years or older, the least deaf group read about as well as the average hearing child at age 10 years, 6 months. The most severely impaired—the most deaf—could read on about the level of an average 8 year, 6 month child.

At the present time there is no evidence to suggest that deaf children in non-English speaking cultures are more proficient in reading than those who have to learn to read English. As a general observation, the limited knowledge of language that is common to the great majority of deaf children is the basic cause of their reading improficiency. Davis and Hardick (1981) note:

The development of good reading skills . . . depends on the development of good language skills. The two cannot be separated, and under optimal conditions they are sequentially learned. As a general rule, severely hearing-impaired children do not exhibit sufficient knowledge of language to insure a basis for the normal development of reading skills. They are expected to learn to read without extensive experience with basic psycholinguistic skills and to use reading as a means of increasing linguistic knowledge from the beginning. With these facts in mind, it would be foolish to expect these children to be able to read as well as their peers. (pp. 282–283)

Approaches to Teaching Reading to the Deaf

Unless the deficits in language knowledge are significantly remediated before reading is formally introduced or language skills are established concurrently with reading, the low level of reading ability is likely to prevail. It is unfortunate that most reading instruction with the deaf is based on assumptions that are appropriate for hearing children. Some concessions are made for "writing down" the content to easier levels and to token awareness of limited knowledge of language. Special instruction, methods that logically are related to visual language, are just beginning to have an impact. "The methods would have to take into account whatever form of visual language the child had internalized prior to the beginning of the reading process" (Quigley & Paul, 1984, p. 138).

I suggest as an alternative an approach that provides a basic functional vocabulary along with grammatic constructions in visual form (illustrations and associated print and, if possible, signed language). Such an approach should be in keeping with our present knowledge of language acquisition in normal hearing children. (*Reading for Meaning: An Illustrated Language Acquisition Program* (Eisenson, 1984b) is such an approach. *Reading Milestones* (Quigley & King, 1984) is a program for the deaf that "systematically introduces increasingly difficult syntactic structures and vocabulary.")

The most widely used sign system—The American Sign Language (ASL)—has a "grammar" of its own that does not parallel the grammatic feature of conventional English grammar. Davis and Hardick (1981, p. 80) provide the following examples of differences between spoken English and ASL:

Spoken English	*ASL*
I was tired when I got home last night.	Yesterday night arrive home tired.
I haven't eaten yet.	Eat late, me.

Following are other examples of differences between conventional spoken English sentences and ASL "equivalents."

Spoken English	*ASL*
Who is that man?	Man who
I went fishing yesterday.	Yesterday fishing I + sign for *finish* to indicate a past event.

The recently devised sign systems that incorporate basic syntactic constructions may provide the foundations for reading that are not inherent in ASL. Among the syntactic sign systems are *Signed English* (Bornstein, 1974) and *Signing Exact English: SEE II* (Gustafson, Pfetzinger, & Azwalkow, 1972). Reports indicate that deaf children taught with syntactic sign systems lag behind the hearing by from 2 to 6 years in their language development. However, the pattern and type of constructions that they acquire are similar to those of hearing children. For a review of studies on sign systems and language development see Quigley and Paul (1984, Chapter 3).

A visual approach to reading—a "starter" for preschool children—is provided in Beatrice Hart's *Teaching Reading to Deaf Children* (1978). Another publication along this line is Bornstein and Saulnier, *The Signed English Starter* (1984). Both of these starter programs are efforts to provide a basic, functional sign "vocabulary" and a systematic progression of the grammatical marker forms that normal hearing children usually have under control by age 3. These "obligatory" morphemes, 14 in all, are markers on words that indicate verb tense endings, auxiliaries, and contracted forms. Because of their importance, they are presented in Table 9-1.

In Chapter Ten we will consider alternate approaches in more detail and provide a rationale for the selected approaches.

TABLE 9-1

FOURTEEN "OBLIGATORY" MORPHEMES (SUFFIXES AND
FUNCTION WORDS) AND THEIR USUAL ORDER
OF ACQUISITION BY CHILDREN

1. Present progressive -ing	Ongoing action	Joe is eating lunch.
2. Preposition: in	Containment	The cookie is in the box.
3. Preposition: on	Support	The cookie is on the box.
4. Plural: -s	Number (more than one)	The birds flew away.
5. Past irregular: e.g., went, ran	The event took place earlier (before the time of the speaker's utterance)	The boy went away. The boy ran away.
6. Possessive: -s	Possession	The girl's dress is red.
7. Uncontracted form of the verb to be (copula): e.g., are, was	Plural number; past tense (earlier in time)	These are cookies. It was a cat. It was on the tree.
8. Articles: the, a	Definite and indefinite article	Bob has the stick. Bob has a stick.
9. Past regular: -ed	Event happened earlier in time	Tom jumped (over) the fence.
10. Third person regular: -s	Third person, present action	He walks fast.
11. Third person irregular: e.g., has, does	Present state (situation) Ongoing action (third person)	He has a ball. She does the cooking.
12. Uncontracted auxiliary be: e.g., is, were	Ongoing action; past action	Bob is eating. They were fishing.
13. Contracted form of to be: e.g., -'s, -'re	State of being (existence)	It's a kitty. We're at home.
14. Contracted auxiliary of be: e.g., -'s, -'re	Time: An ongoing action	He's going. They're eating lunch.

Note: Table is based on the research of R. Brown and Associates (1973) and adaptations from Clark and Clark (1977, p. 345). Reprinted by permission.

CHAPTER TEN

Alternative Approaches for Children at High Risk for Failure

I am a Bear of Very Little Brain, and long words Bother me.

Alexander A. Milne, *Winnie the Pooh*, Chapter 4

Probably the best alternative approach for children who are at high risk for failure in the light of family history of reading and learning disabilities is to postpone formal instruction in reading until at least age 7. The reasons for this are considered in Chapter Six. Age 7 is the first year of formal instruction in the Scandinavian countries, Finland, and the Soviet Union, where the reported incidence of reading disability is no more than 5 percent. As noted earlier, reading disability in the United States, Canada, and Great Britain is at least 20 percent. In these countries reading readiness is introduced in the kindergarten grade and formal instruction usually at age 6, when children are in the first grade. By age 7 many children have already experienced failure in reading with consequences that go far beyond this area of difficulty.

However, if we continue to ignore evidence that waiting a year or more in individual cases may be helpful rather than detrimental, that an added year or more of neurological maturation is the best preventive measure against early failure, then we should introduce reading through alternative approaches to conventional orthography. Such approaches should include maximal visual illustrations and, at least at the outset, a minimum of alphabetic print (conventional orthography). Optimally, a visual illustration program should introduce the child or any other beginner or "second starter" to the principle of a sequence of visual representations—an order or grammar—comparable to those of conventional written (print) systems. This, in turn, should be in keeping with normal grammatical acquisitions in language learning at the stages

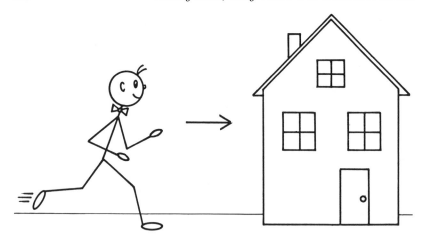

FIGURE 10–1. Possible Rebus representations for "I run home."

when children become aware of how words are put together in making statements of two or more words.

THE REBUS APPROACH

A *rebus* is a pictorial representation of a word or a phrase that is intended to suggest meaning. In the Rebus Approach, symbols that are not directly representational but are so frequently used that their intended meanings can be assumed or readily taught are also employed. Such symbols include arrows (→, ↑, ↓), plus and minus and equal signs (+, −, =), and the letter *s* as a plural or tense indicator. "A bird flies" may be represented by ∿ s; "a boy sits," by 👤 s.

The Peabody Rebus Reading Program (Woodcock & Clark, 1969) was developed to simplify the initial stage of reading for children who might have difficulty with conventional orthography. Printed words are gradually introduced to replace the pictures (pictograms) and so move the beginning reader toward conventional print.

It is possible for a teacher to illustrate a child's sentence, such as "I run home," by rebus characters such as those in Figure 10-1.

The sentence, "I run home," may be used as a specific example (token) of a type of grammatical construction—subject-verb-object or agent-action-noun, and other tokens of the same basic construction may be provided to produce the sentences "I run [to the] store," "I run [to the] school," "I run to the park," etc. These additional tokens will help to establish the notion of a grammatical construction type, first entirely through pictograms and eventually through conventional orthography.

BLISSYMBOLICS (BLISS SYMBOLS)

Blissymbolics was devised by Charles K. Bliss as an international communication system. The Blissymbolic system has been adapted for use as an introduction to reading, as well as a representational approach for communication by persons who cannot speak intelligibly.

Blissymbolics is considerably more sophisticated than the Rebus method. A recent publication, *Blissymbols for Use* (Hehner, 1983), includes a "dictionary" of more than 1,400 symbols. Some of the symbols are "conventionally" representational but not as pictographic as the Rebus characters. For example, *tree* is represented by ⋏, *bird* by ⋎, and child by ⚦. Most of the Bliss symbols are more arbitrary and abstract, constructed according to a system of lines—arcs, wavy lines, and straight lines—in various positions and arrangements. A *gathering* is represented by ⋇, *ear* by ◡, *listen* by ◠, and *to love* by ♡. The statement "I love my mommy," in Bliss symbols may be represented by ⊥ 1♡ (my) ⚦ .

The same construction type can be used with substitutions, such as *daddy, doggy, sister, brother*, etc., in the last position to produce a number of examples (tokens) of the basic grammatical construction. Thus the child is given an opportunity to generalize, if necessary with the help of the teacher, and so become aware of how words (initially pictographs) are arranged to produce statements. Similarly, substitutions may be made in the first position to produce statements such as "You love my daddy," "He loves my mommy," etc.

ADAPTING THE BLISSYMBOLICS

By associating Bliss symbols with printed words, a basic vocabulary and basic grammatical constructions can be taught through a visual-to-visual approach. Beyond the limit of three to four symbols and associated words, Blissymbolics may become too complicated for beginning readers. However, as an introduction and as an alternate to alphabetic print reading at the outset, and by associating the Bliss symbols with conventional orthography, Blissymbolics has its merits. Compared with the Rebus approach, Bliss symbols are more difficult to learn (Clark, 1981). The likely reason for this is that the Rebus characters are essentially pictographs and easily recognizable, while Bliss symbols are more abstract and not as directly representational and therefore need to be learned.

AN ILLUSTRATED LANGUAGE ACQUISITION PROGRAM: READING FOR MEANING

The approach in *Reading for Meaning: An Illustrated Language Acquisition Program (ILAP)*(Eisenson, 1984b) establishes a relationship between decoding for meaning at the outset, rather than one that requires an intermediate step of transcoding from a visual code into speech sounds so that meaning may emerge. The contents of ILAP— *the reading for meaning approach*—include words, phrases, and sentences, each with related picture-illustrations. The association of pictures drawn to provide visual representations of the printed words makes it possible for a child to bypass sound-making (phoneticizing) as an intermediate step between sight and meaning. The populations of children previously identified as at high risk for reading failure (Chapter Nine) require this alternative approach in the beginning stages of learning to read. Those who have already experienced failure by the so-called phonetic approach deserve an opportunity to learn to read by an alternative approach.

Rationale

The underlying assumption for the approach in ILAP is that most of the children who are at high risk for reading failure are *brain different* in basic brain "circuitry." In most instances, they are delayed in the maturation of the "circuitry" that is needed for the integration of the visual, articulatory, and auditory events that are involved in reading.

A second assumption is that the children who are at high risk for reading failure, and especially those who are identified as dyslexic, are less proficient in the knowledge of their language, and particularly of grammar, than we might expect on the basis of cognitive indicators other than those for reading and writing. The approach in ILAP emphasizes the awareness that reading is a language-based skill. Accordingly, knowledge of language—vocabulary, syntax, and meaning—is provided in every one of the five Levels of the program.

Content and Organization of ILAP

The content of ILAP has five Levels, with content assigned according to research data on normal language development generated at Stanford University and other institutions concerned with the study of child language. The Levels progressively include vocabulary items and grammatical constructions that normal children learn to understand and use from about 12 to 48 months of age. At age 4, most children have a considerable amount of their grammatical knowledge under control. That is, they will organize and produce their statements in keeping with the speech of the adults in their environment, even though in many instances such speech is "ungrammatical." Most children continue to gain in their knowledge of grammar well into their secondary school years. The content of ILAP is sufficient to prepare children for reading from the first to the third grades.

The selection of words, expecially in the first three Levels, are ones that are most frequently used in American-English that are also picturable. Examples of selected content are provided in the figures that will follow.

WHERE (AT WHICH LEVEL) TO BEGIN THE ILAP PROGRAM

Where to begin the teaching of this program should be determined by the child's knowledge of English, and particularly by his or her understanding of the meanings of multiword statements. The assumption, of course, is that the child is exposed to a sufficient amount of spoken language that is grammatically correct.

A sample of 50 to 100 of a child's "free" utterances may supply this information. If this sampling is not easy to obtain—many children become remarkably silent when we want them to talk—more formal means of learning what the child understands of grammatical constructions may be necessary. Formal testing procedures are described by Eisenson (1984a).

Another approach, considerably less formal and less anxiety producing and directly related to ILAP, is to use selected items for screening purposes. For Levels I and II, each tenth item—10, 20, etc.—may be used in a "Show me which picture means. . . ." The child is directed (taught to point) to the correct one of three illustrations for the given statement. (For deaf children, this may be done through signing.) Tentatively, we may assume that if the child is correct in response to the selected test items, those that are intermediate are also understood. This assumption, of course, is itself subject to teacher test and modification. When the child fails with three successive items, we have a baseline as to where to begin with the program. It might be prudent to drop back several items in the sequence of presentations to enhance success in learning.

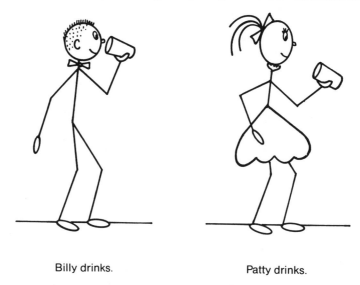

Billy drinks.   Patty drinks.

FIGURE 10–2a. Constructions for noun plus verb (agent-action).

When the child succeeds with a Level, has learned what he or she has been taught, screening for the next Level is in order. This is done so that the teacher may determine what the child has learned about language that was not teacher-taught. The teacher should accept evidence of nondirectly taught knowledge of language as a compliment to his or her teaching.

Level I

Children who are at Level I in normal language development are just beginning to put words together in their spoken utterances. Although they may understand the significance of grammatical markers in the speech they hear, they are not likely to use such features in their own speech. In effect, their speech is agrammatic. Their statements are usually limited to no more than three words. Most children are likely to begin putting words together in sequences such as *Boy run; Doggy bow-wow; Billy drink*. These are noun plus action word (agent-action) constructions. Usually they are followed by action word plus noun combinations (action-agent) such as *Eat banana; Kick ball*. At the upper end of Level I the number of words per utterance usually increases to three or four, so we may get *Look in Tom wagon; Ride in mommy car*.

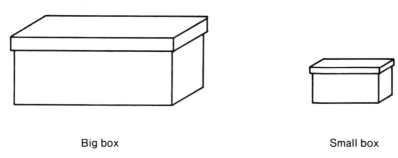

Big box   Small box

FIGURE 10–2b. Contrast: Big vs. small.

Level II

At Level II most children increase the length of their utterances, according to need, from three to four or more words. They also reveal more awareness of the grammatical marker word endings to indicate verb tense, plural, and possessive. They also use the articles *a* and *the* and other small relating words such as *and,* *to* and *for.* At Level II most children who are normal in language development are able to change the order of words to ask questions such as "Is Bobby pulling the wagon?" and answer by "Yes [or No], Bobby is pulling the wagon," or "No, Bobby

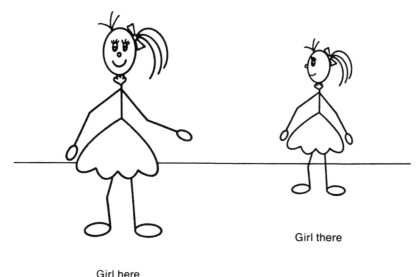

Girl there

Girl here

FIGURE 10–2c. Illustration to establish *here* vs. *there* (noun plus location word).

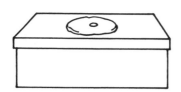
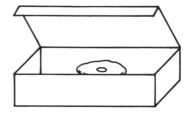

The cookie is <u>on</u> the box.   The cookie is <u>in</u> the box.

Figure 10–2d. Constructions and illustrations for *on* and *in*.

is not pulling the wagon." They can also ask questions beginning with *wh* words such as *where* and *what* to produce "Where is baby?" or the contracted form "Where's baby?" and "What is that?" or "What's that?"

The awareness and use of conventional features of grammar and increase in length of utterances are continued characteristics of normal language development. Both attention span and insights into the conventions of how words are arranged to produce statements and ask questions are associated with these advances. The ability to deal with events that are not objectively in view is probably related to asking *where* and *what* questions.

Level III

Children who are at the Level III stage of language development show an increasing awareness of conventional grammatical features (grammatical markers) in their understanding and production of speech. Articles—*a* and *the*—and the *s* as plural as well as a present tense indicator and as a marker for possessive are reflected in their use of language. Overall, Level III usage tells us that the child has progressed from early child language to adult language. The following illustrated constructions are examples of Level III language. (See Figures 10-3a and 10-3b.)

Level IV

At Level IV in language development, normal children understand and produce sentences that are fully adult in grammatical construction. However, this does not imply that they necessarily understand or have full control of the grammar (syntax) of their language. (Level V will take them to almost average adult proficiency in syntax.) What is implied is

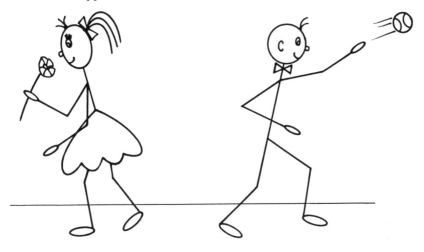

Sally smells flower.   Bobby throws ball.

FIGURE 10–3a. Construction and illustration for noun-verb-object (agent-action-noun).

that if the context of spoken language is not beyond the child's experience, direct or vicarious, and the constructions neither too long nor too complex, comprehension may be assumed. Similarly, in written material, the content does not need to be simplified in regard to grammatical constructions. This does not suggest that the child is ready for future

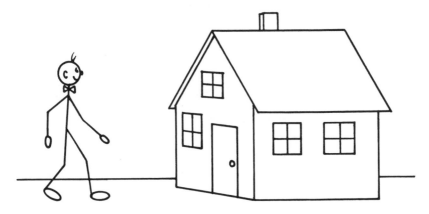

FIGURE 10–3b. Construction and illustration for "Where is the man going?" and answer, "The man is going to the house."

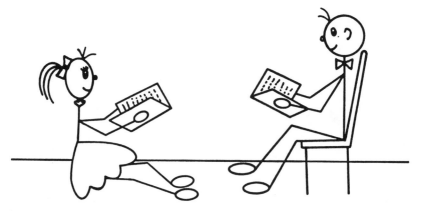

FIGURE 10–4a. Construction and illustration for "They are reading books."

subjunctive statements such as "If I were to . . ." or be certain of the meaning of "John told Bill he's going to the movies." Many 10-year-olds are not certain whether it is John or Bill who will be going to the movies. There is still much to be learned beyond Levels IV and V that cannot be directly taught but may be acquired in the process of learning to read and to enjoy what is available for reading.

The illustrations of constructions that follow indicate some of the advances in grammatical knowledge that characterize Level IV achievements. Highly important among the advances are the understanding

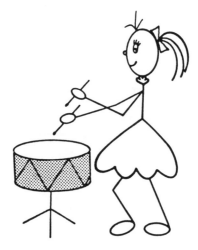

FIGURE 10–4b. Construction and illustration for "A girl is playing a drum."

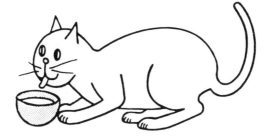

FIGURE 10–4c. Construction and illustration for "What is the kitty doing?" and answer, "Kitty is drinking the milk."

and use of the interrogative words *why, how, whose,* and *which.* Two of these will be included in the illustrated constructions.

Level V

Much that children learn beyond Level IV is about how adults arrange their words to say or write their sentences so that their meanings will be understood and their intentions attained. Somehow most children learn that there is a difference in meaning in such sentences as:

1. Do you want a cookie?
2. Don't you want a cookie?
3. You want a cookie, don't you?
4. You do want a cookie, don't you?

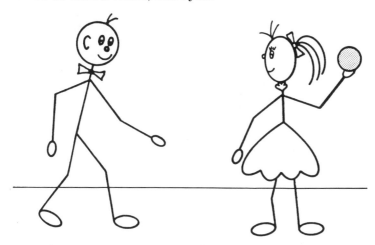

FIGURE 10–4d. Construction and illustration for "She is going to throw the ball."

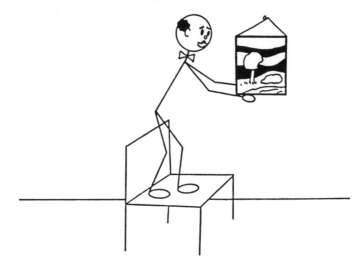

FIGURE 10–5a. Construction and illustration for "The man hangs a picture on the wall."

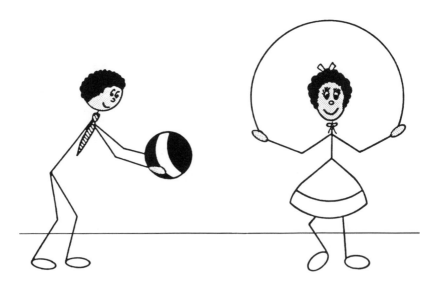

FIGURE 10–5b. Construction and illustration for "Patty would like to jump rope." "Bobby would not like to jump rope."

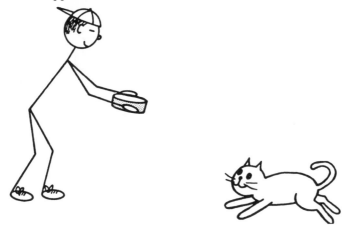

FIGURE 10–5c. Construction and illustration for question, "Why does the kitty run to Dan?" and answer, "The kitty runs to Dan for milk."

Usually, after age 3, a great majority of children say what they need to say in the most effective way according to specific situations. They choose and construct their sentences to bring out not only the surface meaning but also the intention that goes along with the meaning. Those who learn this have learned *linguistic pragmatics* (situational semantics). A minority of children as well as adults lack this knowledge and skill—the art of pragmatics applied to language. This lack is likely to be

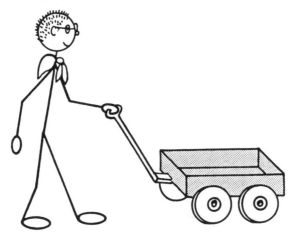

FIGURE 10–5d. Construction and illustration for interrogative *whose:* "Whose_wagon is this?" and answer, "This is Tom's wagon."

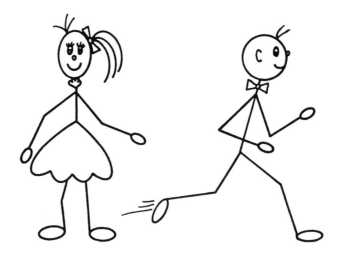

FIGURE 10–6a. Construction and illustration for contracted negative form of *will not* (*won't*). This is a modal (auxiliary) construction that in this instance constitutes a noun plus a modal negative verb: "The girl doesn't run." English modal (auxiliary) verbs include *can, dare, do, may, must, need, shall,* and *will.*

carried over to reading and, of course, to writing. Frankly, I do not believe that such nuances of meaning and appreciation of intentions can be directly taught. Some children may be delayed but will learn linguistic pragmatics through increased exposure, mostly by observing how key adults talk to one another to get what they want through subtleties in language usage. A few, even when they are adult in years, may never quite attain this skill.

In Level V we have a series of constructions that most children who have mastered Level IV are likely to learn without direct teaching. But a few may not. The teacher-clinician can use Level V construction examples as a screening device to determine which of the constructions the child understands and so need not be directly taught, and which do need to be taught in this introductory program for beginning readers.

There is much that children with normal intellectual potential continue to learn and employ in their own productions that cannot possibly be taught. Some children "take off" and learn by leaps and bounds once they become language-prone. Others acquire knowledge about language more slowly and continue to need considerable direct teaching. Children who are identified as aphasic and probably most deaf children need continued direct teaching, regardless of possible grade placement.

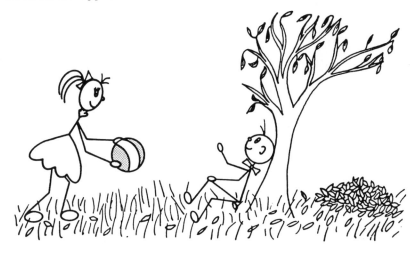

FIGURE 10–6b. Construction and illustration for negative modal as in "The boy won't play."

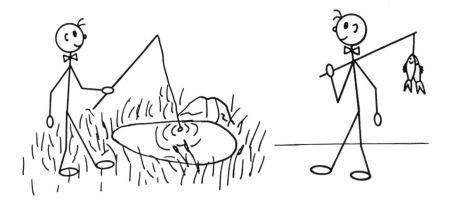

The boy is fishing.   The boy was fishing.

FIGURE 10–6c. Ongoing action vs. past action.

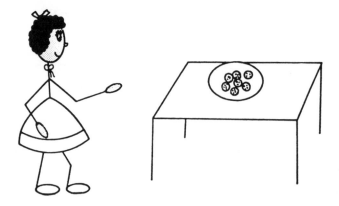

FIGURE 10–6d. Question plus negative modal: "Can't Patty eat the cookies?"

Even normal 10-year-olds have some way to go in their understanding of the differences between "Ask him to go" and "Tell him to go." In context, these differences are not always clear. In good writing, they should be clear. However, these relatively advanced teachings are beyond the scope of Reading for Meaning: An Illustrated Language Acquisition Program.

CHAPTER ELEVEN

Higher Levels of Learning in Reading

by Elise Trumbull Estrin, Ed.D.*

Reading can be compared to the performance of a symphony orchestra. This analogy illustrates three points. First, like the performance of a symphony, reading is a holistic act. In other words, while reading can be analyzed into subskills such as discriminating letters and identifying words, performing the subskills one at a time does not constitute reading. Reading can be said to take place only when the parts are put together in a smooth, integrated performance. Second, success in reading comes from practice over long periods of time, like skill in playing musical instruments. Indeed, it is a lifelong endeavor. Third, as with a musical score, there may be more than one interpretation of a text. The interpretation depends upon the background of the reader, the purpose for reading, and the context in which reading occurs.

Becoming a Nation of Readers: The Report of the Commission on Reading (1985).

The concept of reading as a process of deriving meaning from print, rather than simply deciphering words or transcoding from a written to an oral form, has already been well established in this book. We emphasize that syntactic and semantic processes are more important in mature reading than simple "phoneticizing" to identify a word. (Of course,

---

*Dr. Elise Trumbull Estrin, a psycholinguist and expert on reading, is concerned with helping children and adults to learn to read in depth. Her chapter will provide information on where to go and how to get there to learn how to read with understanding and skills that are not usually taught in most school programs. This information is intended not only for those who were initially at high risk for failure, and many of whom continue to be reluctant readers, but also for good readers who can become even better at the reading game. These "good" readers may still be in school, possibly even at the college level, or may be finished with their formal education. Reading for depth of meaning and reading for pleasure are both reasonable goals for most persons of moderate or above-average intelligence.

phonetic analysis skills are also useful for those who can acquire them, particularly in the early stages of learning to read.) What I shall do in this chapter is discuss some of the high-level intellectual or cognitive aspects of the reading process and how knowledge of these cognitive aspects can be used by the teacher to help readers to improve their strategies for reading with understanding.

Cognitive functions (cognition) refer to learning and learning how we learn to know (gaining knowledge and insights). Language as the major instrument of learning is obviously also a major form of cognition.

READING AS A CONSTRUCTIVE ACTIVITY

Reading and listening are both *active language processes*. They have in common a basic need for proficiency in oral language, or in the case of most of the deaf, of sign language. However, there are important differences in the aspects of the written and spoken language systems and the processes by which we receive and send meaningful messages.

Actually, the written language medium is quite different from the spoken. Many of the cues to meaning that are present in face-to-face speaking are missing in writing. Most spoken language is in the form of conversation, and that is what children have experienced as they approach the age of learning to read. In conversation, children have the benefit of such cues as facial expressions, of pauses to express emphasis or allow time for comprehension, and gestures (which may help with understanding of pronouns, spatial references, and topics about people or objects near at hand). Unless we are talking to ourselves, conversation requires at least two participants. Clarifications can be made by asking questions or showing lack of understanding nonverbally—a shake of the head, a quizzical look. The turn-taking nature of conversation allows for checks on comprehension and for keeping both speakers involved.

In learning to read, a child has to make the best guesses possible about meaning without being able directly to question the author as to purpose. If attention or interest wanes, the author cannot leap forward and grab the reader by the shoulders or glare at him. All of these kinds of differences between the two modalities need to be appreciated in order to grasp the nature of the task that readers face.

Most reading theorists now believe strongly that reading is a highly complex process in which meaning is *constructed* in an interaction between reader and text. The reader uses his or her own knowledge of the world, of language, and of how texts tend to be structured to determine the meaning of what he reads. Good readers have well-developed strategies for bringing all of these kinds of knowlege to bear in order to understand what they read. From this point of view, reading might well be characterized as a problem-solving task, calling upon a number of different skills and sources of knowledge.

As discussed in Chapter Four, readers do need to make use of their oral language knowledge. Despite the differences between speaking and reading, there is considerable overlap between oral and written language in vocabulary and syntax. Good readers use their knowledge of vocabulary and syntax to figure out what is on the page. Using their syntactic knowledge, they tend to read in phrases rather than word-by-word. They are quicker than poor readers at matching written words to their oral forms.

Some studies have suggested that poor readers actually have inferior oral syntatic skills. However, it appears that the biggest problem is that in most cases improficient readers do not use the oral language knowledge they do have when confronted with print. For some reason, they cannot or do not make this knowledge available or accessible for use in reading. This is not entirely surprising, for speaking is something most people do (most of the time) without conscious intellectual effort. All too often, it is virtually automatic. In reading, this automatic, tacit language knowledge needs to become more conscious, or at least accessible. It can then be applied to a new modality—language in visual form. This different (and relatively new, historically) form of language is a *secondary* symbol system derived from the oral, or *primary*, symbol system. Unlike oral language learning, acquisition of reading skill usually requires formal, explicit instruction. Most people do not learn to read simply by being exposed to books and having stories read to them. An important part of instruction is showing the learner just how written language is related to oral language and encouraging him or her to formalize or make conscious the oral language knowledge he or she possesses. Unfortunately, not many reading programs do this with much insight or success.

COMPREHENSION PROCESSES

Literal and Inferential Comprehension

Ellen Gagné, an educational psychologist, emphasizes the difference between two basic kinds of reading comprehension: the literal and the inferential (Gagné, 1985). Literal comprehension occurs when a reader accurately puts word meanings together to form meaningful state-ments. Inferential comprehension occurs when the reader goes beyond the meaning explicitly stated and integrates, summarizes, or elaborates upon what is read. Literal comprehension may be sufficient for reading such things as timetables and simple instructions, but it is likely that even in these cases some inferential comprehension is necessary. Cer-tainly, reading of literature and of "content area" texts (science, social studies, etc.) requires inferential comprehension. Poor readers, as might be expected, show greater deficits in inferential than literal comprehension. Let us look more closely at what kinds of inferences readers need to be able to make and what is entailed in inferential comprehension.

Although we are rarely conscious that we are making inferences, all of us do so constantly in our conversation, in reading, and in all activities of daily life. Our common knowledge about the world allows us to make inferences—logical or reasonable assumptions based on information that has been explicitly presented to us in one form or another. For example, in reading the sentence, "She unlocked the door," most per-sons would readily infer the presence of a key of some sort. More tangential inferences can also be made. The door probably has hinges; the key is probably made of metal; the person doing the unlocking has the use of at least one hand. These more peripheral inferences probably will not occur unless a teacher asks for them or they come to have some importance later on in the text. Note that an inference must be plausible but need not be a logical requirement or conclusion. The door *might* have some unusual construction; a key *could* be made of heavy plastic; a disabled person or someone with hands full *could* use her mouth rather than her hand to manipulate a key.

Components of Inferential Comprehension in Reading

Integration is the process of relating ideas or propositions to each other, either within sentences, between sentences, or between one part of the text and another. For example, readers must keep track of pronouns and the nouns to which they refer. The following is a sample of text from *The Little, Brown Book of Anecdotes*, by Clifton Fadiman: "One of (Joseph) Turner's most famous and popular pictures was his painting of the fire that destroyed the Old House of Parliament in 1834. It is remarkable for its evocation of an immensely complex scene caught at a moment of high drama" (Fadiman, 1985, p. 553). A reader needs to be able to determine that the "it" which begins the second sentence refers to the painting mentioned in the first sentence. It would be easy to make a false start in comprehending this sentence because in the phrase "It is remarkable" the "it" often does not have a clear antecedent reference. A competent reader will readily keep track of pronouns across sentences, but poor readers often have difficulty with even this kind of integration. As a result, they may lose track of which characters are doing what actions, or—as could happen with the sentences cited—fail to grasp what is being described.

Integration also requires relating sentences that are not related on the surface. For example in the pair of sentences that follows, an inference must be made to understand their underlying relationships: "The alarm clock rang. Liz jumped out of bed." We infer that the alarm had been set to awaken Liz at a certain time and that she needed to arise at this time, perhaps to get ready for work or some other appointment. Again, poorer readers are much less proficient than good readers at making these cross-sentence connections, and as a result their comprehension suffers.

As can be well imagined, the problem becomes more serious when ideas must be integrated from one part of the text to another. Even in simple narratives, children must keep track of earlier details in order to understand later events. In *The Tale of Benjamin Bunny*, by Beatrix Potter (1904), we are told on page 22 that Peter's clothes are on a scarecrow in Mr. McGregor's garden. Three pages of text and several pictures later, Benjamin Bunny suggests that he and Peter retrieve the clothes. There is no reminder of what happened to them or where they are, but children are expected to integrate the two pieces of information. Of course, more advanced texts (junior high school history texts, for example) require more abstract kinds of integration involving ideas such as human rights, or international policies.

Summarizing is the process of developing an overall mental outline for the passage one is reading. The way the passage is written (the text structure, which will be discussed in more detail shortly) should help the reader to compose this outline. A true outline has a hierarchy of levels. There are top-level headings with subheadings below and items within those subheadings. Proficient readers show evidence of summarizing or making such hierarchical mental outlines as they read, and they are more likely than poor readers to be able to distinguish the most important information from less important details in what they have read. They are apparently actively organizing (although not entirely consciously) what they read as they go along and so are able to recall it.

Elaboration entails drawing on one's prior knowledge while reading, in effect facilitating understanding of the text by tying new information to familiar concepts, i.e., what is already known. Elaboration can take the form of activating visual images the reader has on related information, asking questions about the text and how it relates to his or her own experience and beliefs, or drawing comparisons between new concepts and known concepts. Elaboration is integration between text and reader, rather than between parts of the text. Not only do good readers participate in more elaboration, but we know that it is important to comprehension. Investigations by Weinstein, Underwood, Wicker, & Cubberly (1979), Mayer (1980, 1983), and many others have shown that poor readers can improve in comprehension by being shown how to elaborate on what they are reading. We will discuss this process in more detail in the section below on prior knowledge, since it has been shown to be a critical contributor to good comprehension.

Using Prior Knowledge to Construct Meaning

In reading about any topic, a proficient reader will draw upon knowledge he or she already has about the topic to make sense of and evaluate the text at hand. As mentioned above, readers draw heavily on prior knowledge for inferential comprehension. Anderson and Pearson (1984) remind us that knowledge that is already stored is used to interpret new information, and the reader may find either that the new information fits into his or her existing framework (or schema) about the topic or that the framework has to be revised in order to accommodate new facts.

For example, in reading about the restoration of a Botticelli painting in Florence, Italy, the reader might almost unconsciously search his or her memory to recall when Botticelli lived (and thus what kind of paints he used or what state of decay the painting may be in), whether any natural disasters might have contributed to the damage (as happened in floods in certain parts of Italy in the late 1960s), or anything he or she already knows about techniques of restoration. When doing so, the reader is using prior knowledge to elaborate on new concepts.

Tierney and Cunningham (1984) summarize investigations that show that good readers make use of prior knowledge and that young readers and older poor readers do not draw as much on their existing knowledge to help them understand what they read. That is, some readers either do not realize the importance of activating their own knowledge on the topic at hand or are unable to do so. They read passively, expecting all the important material to be on the page. The problem for other readers of any age may be that they do not have much prior knowledge on which to call. They may have no "schema" or set of facts and concepts about the author's subject.

To use the Botticelli example mentioned earlier, many a newspaper reader encountering an article on Botticelli may in fact have very little useful prior knowledge to invoke. Such a reader would have to rely on just what the article provided and might miss some of the implications or inferences that a more knowledgeable person could derive. This is, of course, true for anyone reading about an unfamiliar topic. One person's organizational framework (schema) may vary slightly from another's because of differences in personal experience, but for ordinary topics there will be a great deal of overlap among people in the ways their schemata are organized. Most readers will have a schema for understanding a common activity such as shopping at the grocery store. They have an organized framework that relates the various components of grocery shopping: planning what groceries are needed, perhaps making a list, going to the store, taking a shopping cart and selecting the proper items, paying, and transporting the goods home, where they will be stored in various ways.

It is important for teachers to remember that a young child's schema for any topic cannot be expected to be equivalent to the adult's. We all build our schemata from experience, revising them unconsciously as we have new experiences. Children, of course, have a much more limited reservoir of experience on which to draw. They may be lacking important knowledge of components of various schemata and of how those components are related. Young readers may not know, for example, that at some grocery stores there are people who will carry packages out to the parking lot. At times these missing pieces of knowledge can cause gaps in reading comprehension.

It is clear that much of the information readers need in order to comprehend what they read does not reside in the text but in their own heads. (We read with our brains by way of our eyes.) In fact, authors count on the fact that readers do not have to be told everything. A shared knowledge base—at least about ordinary events and relationships in the world—is presumed. But obviously, not all readers of the same text will be able to make exactly the same inferences, since ability to make inferences is based largely on prior knowledge, and readers' experiences vary. If, however, the reader can activate his or her prior knowledge—whatever it is—comprehension will improve. At the end of this chapter we will offer several suggestions as to how teachers and parents can foster this activation.

Using the Structure of Text in Comprehension

Interwoven with the issue of the content of written material and the way a reader schematizes that content in his or her own mind is the matter of how the text itself is structured. On one level, there may be visible cues to what is important in the passage (chapter, story, etc.). Writers and editors often use headings, bold print, italics, and other graphic devices to elucidate relationships among parts of a text, particularly in textbooks or scholarly articles. For example, most important or top-level concepts are in larger or darker print. A list may include "bullets" or numbers that highlight important points. (See pages 36, 47, 76 for such listings.)

At a somewhat more abstract level, there is usually an overall narrative or expository structure to a piece of writing. For good comprehension, readers need to make use of knowledge of text structure (as has been demonstrated by researchers including Meyer, 1975, 1977, 1985; and Stein & Glenn, 1979). In reading a narrative, it is very helpful to have a sense of the standard format. Most narratives have a relatively predictable format and set of components. A setting will be presented early on in the story; there will be characters and some kind of plot that typically entails a problem and its solution, with various steps in between.

Many children have been exposed to bedtime stories often enough to be able to anticipate the structure of narrative, thereby facilitating comprehension in early reading. Some, however, may not have been read to enough to have internalized a concept of story. These children are more likely to have comprehension problems when they begin to read.

Unfortunately, early reading texts do not always use good story structure in their selections. In an effort to keep vocabulary simple and representative of certain spelling patterns, the writers of beginning texts often produce stories with very little meaning and virtually *no* structure. In such instances, teachers usually complement the reading program with language experience activities that require the child to draw on knowledge of story structure by producing his or her own stories. Reading to children in class from well-formed stories can also compensate for lack of structure in beginning reading texts. A good reading series will, however, have real stories that engage the child, and all the research evidence strongly suggests that the child who has been read to a great deal during the preschool years is likely to be the successful reader in the school years.

In addition to reading stories, children have to learn how to read what is called "expository" text. Expository writing consists of description, commentary, or explanation. Typically, young children encounter expository texts in the form of descriptions of animals or of kinds of transportation, discussions of how people live in communities or of life in other lands (social studies topics), explanations of how to make something such as a paper kite or walkie-takie, or directions for a simple science experiment.

As with narrative or story structure, there are predictable formats for expository writing. Directions, recipes, and instructions for science experiments are in the form of sequences or steps in a process. Descriptions of animals may be in the form of what Stanford University professor Robert Calfee (Calfee & Curley, 1984) has called a "topical net," with the animal as topic and various details or facts (what it eats, where it lives, what it looks like) used to build a description. More advanced science writing may take the form of a hierarchy in which elements are assigned to different levels (animals, vertebrates, mammals, primates, etc.). Another useful kind of text organization is the matrix in which several topics are treated in light of a number of categories (reptiles, mammals, and birds described according to their mode of reproduction, body coverings, etc.). Later on the reader may be exposed to forms of argument, but these are not likely to be encountered in primary texts.

In the same way that awareness of story structure aids comprehension, awareness of expository structure helps readers figure out how pieces of information are related within a passage. A reader who is familiar with such formats as description, sequence, hierarchy, and matrix is more likely to understand what the author of an expository passage is trying to communicate than one who does not. Research has shown that poor readers do not make use of the text structure; rather they tend to recall details in a listlike way instead of in relation to each other. In a study of ninth-graders, using two different kinds of expository text structure, Meyer, Brandt, and Bluth (1980) found that about three-fourths of good readers, about one-half the number of average readers, and *less* than one-fourth of poor readers used the text structure to help them remember the passages. Again, we have a strong argument for reading to children from many different kinds of books at an early age. By so doing, we prepare them for the variety of texts they will need to comprehend.

Self-Monitoring Activities in Reading

There is another set of skills which good readers increasingly rely on as they mature. Not only do good readers draw inferences, bring to bear their prior knowledge, and make use of the text structure; they perform a number of objective, so-called "executive" functions to monitor and control their reading. Ann L. Brown, a cognitive psychologist at the Center for the Study of Reading (University of Illinois, Urbana-Champaign) has written a great deal on this subject. She says that readers need to keep one eye on the content of what they are reading and the other on their own learning processes. They need to ask themselves whether they are doing what they need to do to understand. First, they set goals when they read, and they use different strategies to attain different goals. For example, if the goal is to learn as many details as possible, they go through the text with a fine-toothed comb, as it were. If they are reading to gain broad concepts or a general idea of what is contained in a chapter, they focus on headings and topic sentences and skim over details.

Second, good readers monitor their success as they go along, checking periodically to see whether they have understood what they have read and whether they have met their goal. If not, they may reread certain portions of the text or modify their strategies in an effort to improve comprehension. Technically, these skills are referred to as "*meta*cognitive," because they function beyond or outside the basic comprehension skills, as a kind of outer layer surrounding all the other skills.

Good readers also have well-developed "*meta*linguistic" skills, that is, through their knowledge of language, they monitor the language they read. They use their knowledge of language to catch errors. If they misread a word, with a resulting grammatical error, they notice their mistake and look back to clarify what they have read. They also seem to use their linguistic knowledge in context to anticipate upcoming words and phrases and to identify unknown vocabulary. Poor readers are much less successful at goal-setting and at monitoring, both at the level of linguistic errors that result in misunderstandings and more globally at the level of passage comprehension.

Research has shown that less mature readers either do not notice or do not know how to resolve conflicts in comprehension. Since poor readers tend to look like less mature readers in their reading strategies, studies comparing younger with older readers are often used to add to the information pool on underdeveloped reading skills. One study (Harris, Kruithof, Terwogt, and Visser, 1981) showed that younger children (third-graders) generally did not notice an inappropriate sentence in a short story. Children were given a story entitled "John at the Dentist" which contained the sentence, "He sees his hair getting shorter." Only 11% could identify the sentence as being inconsistent with the title.

Sixth-graders in the same study had much greater success—44% could identify the sentence that did not fit.

Interestingly, however, the younger children took longer to read stories inappropriately titled than comparable stories that were correctly titled. This suggests that though the younger readers could not overtly state the problem, they were influenced by it. A study by Garner & Reis (1981) also showed that good readers are more strategic about solving comprehension problems. For example, they know when they should look back within the text they have read to find answers to questions. Students in Grades 4 through 10 were given several paragraphs and questions relating to them. The younger, poor comprehenders who did recognize that they had a comprehension problem failed to look back to find answers (doing so only 9% of the time). The oldest and best readers consistently used a look-back strategy (80%). This is an example of children's recognizing that they have a comprehension problem without knowing how to resolve it.

Other studies (Ryan & Ledger, 1978; Hook and Johnson, 1978; Menyuk & Flood, 1981; among many) have shown that *average* readers are significantly less able than good readers to monitor their own reading for linguistic errors. They are not disturbed by grammatical errors and have difficulty spotting ambiguity. They may not realize that a word or phrase can have more than one meaning and that their first interpretation may not be the correct one. It is clear from these and other studies that poor readers are distinguished from good readers rather consistently by their inability to use monitoring strategies in comprehension.

The Issue of Automaticity

We know that the brain has a limited capacity for attention and short-term memory. That is, at any given time, we can consciously attend to and hold in mind only so many pieces of information. The average person can remember only about seven individual pieces of information at a time unless these pieces can be organized in relation to each other in some meaningful way. (The limitations of the capacity of the brain to attend to on-going events is clearly explained by La Berge & Samuels, 1974.) If we are focused on recalling what sounds a given letter of the alphabet can stand for so as to start to figure out the beginning of a word, we will have less attention to devote to anticipating what might happen later on in the sentence in which that word occurs. If we move very slowly through a sentence, word-by-word, we may forget what happened at the beginning. A good reader quickly recognizes words and chunks them together in meaningful phrases. Certain parts of the reading process have become automatic.

It may be that for many poor readers the tasks of word identification and literal sentence comprehension consume the majority of their energies. They have not become automatic at these tasks. A broader, more planful approach that involves goal-setting, use of different strategies, and monitoring the success of those strategies (i.e., the state of their comprehension), may simply be beyond their attending and memory capacity. What is needed is a more efficient rate of processing. If this is the case, perhaps educational intervention should focus first on helping these students automatize some of their lower-level skills and subsequently to develop such higher-level skills as inferential reasoning, text awareness, and comprehension monitoring.

WHAT PARENTS AND TEACHERS CAN DO TO DEVELOP COGNITIVE ASPECTS OF READING COMPREHENSION

What Parents Can Do

Any adult or older child can help the younger child or disabled reader gain a better chance of developing into a proficient reader by reading to him or her from a variety of kinds of books. This has been said before, but it can hardly be stressed too strongly. The more familiar a reader is with multiple text types, the more awareness he or she can bring to the task of learning to read. Not only does exposure to all kinds of books enhance awareness of text structure, but it gets the potential reader accustomed to extracting information (and entertainment) from a non-conversational source. In addition, it increases the child's knowledge base. Having the child tell original stories or give accounts of daily events also builds a notion of story. In this situation, an adult can gently offer assistance in structuring the telling (by asking questions) if the child falters or leaves out an important link.

To foster integration, summarization, and elaboration (inferential comprehension), adults can check to make sure children understand relationships across sentences by asking questions and eliciting children's comments about the story. Good questions might be, "What does this remind you of?" or "What do you think about what Alice did? Would you do that?" or "Can you tell me the most important things that have happened so far?" or "Can you remember the most important things we have learned about how polar bears live?" It may be necessary to offer some cues such as, "Well, what kind of food do they eat?" Perhaps the most important thing to get across to the potential reader is that reading is an active process in which we use our own ideas and questions to help us understand.

What Teachers Can Do

There are a great many instructional techniques that can be used to help slowly developing readers or those with serious problems (dyslexic readers). Many of these techniques probably benefit good readers as well, although it has been shown extensively in research that good readers generally use these techniques or strategies without a great deal of explicit instruction. What follows here is a summary of activities and techniques that have been successful in increasing growth in the cognitive components of reading. There have been hundreds of studies on these techniques in the last ten years. (For a thorough review, see Tierney and Cunningham, 1984.) Briefly, they include activities for: (1) actually developing background knowledge, (2) helping readers to activate prior knowledge before and during reading, (3) helping readers set goals in reading, (4) providing guidance during reading, and (5) assisting readers through postreading review activities.

Prereading Activities

Vocabulary Development/Activating Prior Knowledge: One way to increase comprehension of passages to be read is to build knowledge of key vocabulary that will be encountered in the passage. An extremely successful approach to this is a brainstorming technique in which the teacher puts a topic on the blackboard and asks students to think of words associated with it. Discussion can ensue about meanings of words and their relationships, and they can be categorized in subtopics. For example, if an upcoming topic in the reading is "transportation," students can supply the terms, while the teacher asks questions about the description and purpose of various vehicles; and they can be sorted according to such categories as "land," "sea," and "air." The teacher can, of course, introduce words the students do not supply.

Another advantage of this activity is that it stimulates use of prior knowledge of a topic, and new concepts can be linked to concepts already known.

Previews, Summaries, and Supplementary Discussion or Reading: Discussion of the topic or story line that children will be reading about has been shown to foster comprehension. As might be expected, discussion that links prior knowledge or children's previous experiences to the story to be read helps to improve inferential comprehension. Brief previews in written form have also been used with some success, particularly if they include additional background knowledge that is not included in the text. They have been most helpful with texts that students find difficult.

Using Advance Organizers: An advance organizer is an activity or material used to prepare the reader for a specific text. There are many kinds of advance organizers, and there is not complete agreement on which are the most useful. That depends on the kind of text, the purpose of the reading, and the age and skills of the reader. A good advance organizer provides the reader with a structure for approaching the text. It could be a series of questions that require integrating information in the text. It has been found that if questions are used, they are most helpful if given before *and* after reading.

At high school level in content area classrooms, a structured overview that essentially outlines the most important concepts and relationships in the text is often used. The story preview mentioned above is really a form of advance organizer. In general, advance organizers do more to facilitate grasping broad concepts and relationships and retaining them over long periods of time than they do to improve short-term memory for details.

Setting Goals in Reading: Studies have shown that students read differently depending on what their goal is. Of course, different goals will be appropriate to different kinds of texts and settings, and good readers seem to be able to set their own goals as well as figure out how to read to satisfy teachers' expectations. Research suggests that it can be useful to set objectives or goals prior to reading, especially if there is a need to read selectively, for example, to satisfy test preparation requirements. Learning-disabled children seem to read with better comprehension if given goals beforehand, but children with attention deficits do not consistently benefit from being given goals.

Activities Done During Reading

Self-Questioning and Teacher Questioning: Students trained to ask themselves comprehension questions as they read have shown increased comprehension, but unless younger students *are* actually trained, they may not have success in formulating useful questions. For younger students, it has been most beneficial to have teacher-prepared questions inserted periodically in the text. If adjunct questions are given to be completed at the end of reading, it may be necessary to remind students to look back through the text to refresh their memory. As we know, less mature readers may fail to use even that simple strategy.

Comprehension Monitoring: Students can also be helped to be aware of the strategies they use to comprehend when reading. One successful training program showed students how to answer questions about text more strategically by determining if the answer was in the text, was to be derived from one's own background knowledge, or was to be derived by relating different concepts in the text to each other (Pearson & Johnson, 1977; Hansen & Pearson, 1983). Many students seem to expect the answer to be explicit in the text only. Such students will not exhibit good inferential comprehension.

Students need to realize that not all of the content of a passage is explicit, and they need to learn how to monitor their comprehension by asking the more general questions, "Did I understand what I just read? If not, what can I do to help myself understand?" For students who do not monitor their comprehension (i.e., who do not seem to realize when they have not understood what they have read), there are activities that can help to develop this monitoring ability. One way to self-check is to write a summary sentence after reading each paragraph. Such summarization itself aids comprehension. Peer interviews, in which two students quiz each other, can be helpful. Both formulating and answering questions help comprehension.

Elaboration Exercises: As was mentioned in the section on inferential comprehension, better comprehension occurs when readers elaborate on what they read by tying new concepts to their existing knowledge. Students can be given tasks that require them to elaborate. The simplest kind of elaboration is association of two words either through a visual image or a sentence. This is helpful for literal comprehension and memory, particularly of items that need to be recalled in a rote fashion, such as parts of the inner ear, stages in cell division, or state capitals.

For inferential comprehension, the reader needs to go beyond the text and actively group new concepts with known ones or make comparisons between some concept in the text and another already in memory. A student might be asked to compare a pet described in a story with his or her own pet, or to add descriptive details that would be plausible for an event in a story. At more advanced levels, a student might be required to construct an analogy to something appearing in the text from personal experience. Telling or writing about personal knowledge that is related to a text topic facilitates inferential processes more than drawing about the same experiences (something young children are often asked to do in school). In general, verbal elaboration is more powerful than visual imagery elaboration.

Teaching Text Structure: There are educators who have shown that children as young as first-grade age can begin to use the structure of text to understand what they read. There are systems for identifying different kinds of texts (narrative and various kinds of exposition), and there is no doubt that good readers use text-structure knowledge. Some teachers will want to investigate these programs. (See references marked with an asterisk.) In the absence of explicit instruction on text structure, students can benefit greatly from being exposed to (being read to or reading themselves) a variety of kinds of texts, beginning in early childhood.

Postreading Activities

Questioning and Review: Teachers can pose the same questions they asked in the prereading phase, something that has been shown to foster inferential comprehension (specifically, integration of material read). Teacher-guided group discussion is generally more useful than student group discussion (without teacher), but both are better than no discussion following reading. Higher-level questions, or those that require thinking about broad concepts and linking them, result in greater and longer-lasting learning. Questions and reviews can, of course, be followed by tests.

Feedback: Teachers should give students immediate feedback about their performance, whether for exercises, in-class questions and discussion, or tests. Students learn more when given feedback, and feedback on errors is more important than feedback on correct performance. Although most teachers recognize the *motivational* importance of giving students positive feedback, they may not realize the *instructional* value of feedback. In fact, negative feedback—information to the student that he or she has not understood something—is extremely important. It is important to the student whose performance is being examined and to other students who are listening. Negative feedback need not be given in a way that embarrasses the student. The teacher can give gentle correction, turning attention away from the student who has erred unless he or she seems ready to revise a response.

A Final Note on Instructional Techniques

The majority of instruction is presented to children without any explanation as to *why* specific tasks are being done. Often when children are asked why they are doing a workbook activity or completing a teacher-designed assignment, they say they do not know or that they are doing it because the teacher told them to. Instruction should include a rationale to students for the activities they are asked to participate in. Even a first-grader can be told that answering questions about a story will help him or her to understand and remember it. Students will use the comprehension techniques they are taught more successfully when they understand how the techniques work and what they do to foster comprehension. Techniques which are both modeled *and* explained by the teacher are better learned and used by students than techniques that are only modeled.

A Case History of a Familial Dyslexic

Despite his early school problems because of his inability to learn to read—Tom R. was identified as a dyslexic child in the third grade—he managed to get through both elementary and high school, was graduated from a California state university, and then earned a graduate degree from an Ivy League university. Despite these achievements, Tom still regards himself as an improficient reader because he cannot readily make full sense out of written language. He does not enjoy reading and rarely reads anything of length for pleasure. His spelling is "approximate" but sufficiently close to the target so that he is usually able to decode his notes. All of this indicates that Tom R. has come a long way from being a nonreader who was once thought to be mentally inadequate if not mentally retarded.

Tom's three year older sister learned to read before she entered the kindergarten grade. His sister walked unaided at 8 months, began to talk intelligibly at 9 months, and was completely toilet-trained by 15 months. She was by all evidence a precocious child with a determined Intelligence Quotient of above 140. From kindergarten on through secondary school, she was consistently among the highest achievers. She won an academic scholarship to a prestigious college.

In sharp contrast, Tom was conspicuously slow in his development. He did not walk until 18 months, was generally awkward, and inclined to bump into anything that was bumpable. Tom "jabbered" unintelligibly until he was almost 30 months of age and was 6 months older before he was toilet-trained. Not only was Tom delayed in starting to speak intelligibly, he also had considerable difficulty in understanding what his sister and his mother said to him.[1] He began to figure them out when he was about age 4. Strangers, except for one aunt, were completely beyond him. Tom complained that they all spoke too fast and said too much at one time. His sister and mother and the special aunt spoke slowly, and almost always about things that were present for him to see. Most of the time his father spoke too quickly to be understood and became impatient when Tom failed to understand. Nor did father make certain that he had his son's attention when he addressed him. Tom's father could not figure out why the boy did usually understand his mother and sister, and assumed that he had a special kind of listening loss and hoped that he would "grow out of it."

At about age 5, Tom began to understand what most members of his family—his aunts and cousins and grandparents—said to him but he complained to his mother that they still talked "funny" and too fast. He still could not follow conversations between grown-ups because they said too much and spoke too fast.

When Tom entered kindergarten, his school difficulties began. He could not sing in tune, he was confused between right and left, he could not keep his place in a line, and frequently bumped into his classmates. He spilled paints and whatever else was spillable. He had difficulty in cutting with scissors because he was left-handed and all of the scissors available to the children were made for those who were right-handed. (Tom's teacher thought him to be "neither-handed.") His difficulty with scissors was partially solved when Tom's mother provided him, with teacher approval, with a pair of left-handed scissors. His crayon work and paste-ons rarely came within the defined borders.[2]

Reading readiness materials were a mystery and a source of frustration. They provided an opportunity for failure to follow directions and to draw lines and fill in spaces that had no meaning for Tom. However, pre-school provided one saving situation. Whenever any games or teaching involved numbers, Tom was first to announce the correct answer. Even here, the situation was not an unmitigated pleasure. The teacher insisted that he, like all other children, was expected to wait until recognized and heard his name called. Tom was rarely able to contain himself that long. Fortunately, his teacher became aware of Tom's "waiting disability" and began to call his name promptly, especially when he remembered to raise his right hand.

In the first grade it became evident that Tom could not associate the alphabet letters with the sound or sounds they were supposed to make. He could not "word call" when presented with cards that had squiggles that represented words that his classmates understood but were a mystery to him. On rare occasions, if he had time to study a card carefully, he could "word call" the card correctly. Tom did best with real words that were associated with pictures. When presented with cards that had just single letters or combinations of letters, Tom found the mystery of sounds the letters are supposed to make completely beyond his grasp. After considerable drill, he made some progress in identifying the names of the letters, and was able to sound a few such as *s* and *p* whose sounds resembled the names of the letters. Although he finally managed to learn a few letter combinations and could guess the sounds he was expected to produce for them, his productions were not consistent. Often he transposed the sounds so that an *sk* came out as *ks* and a *st* as *ts*. The printed word *cat*, unless accompanied by a picture, might be produced as *tac* and *man* as *nam*. Sometimes Tommy self-corrected his error, more likely with a phrase or a short sentence if his production made no sense to him. For example, he might say "I nur. No, I run."

Because of his difficulties in reading, Tommy was first identified as a "slow learner" and probably mentally retarded. His teacher was surprised and his family relieved when the school psychologist, after administering a standardized test of intelligence, reported an IQ of 128, not much below that of his sister. However, the score raised the expectations of his perplexed teacher, who decided that Tommy was either not trying hard enough or was just lazy or, perhaps even worse, was indifferent to her teaching.

Learning to write produced new problems. His spelling seemed to be a random sequence of illegible scrawls. Individual letters were difficult to identify and inconsistent in shape and form. Some appeared to be created for the occasion. He could not copy words from sample so that *pat* might come out as *tap* and *kitty* as *tikty* and *boy* as *yob*. However, if presented with a picture that included a *kitty* and a *boy*, he might well "read" the picture as "Boy and kitty." Overall, however, Tommy's writing resembled his preschool-age "scribble" speech.

Despite his obvious improficiencies, Tommy was promoted through the primary and middle grades. This was partly a result of the school's policy for "social and age-grade promotions" and partly because he did excell in arithmetic and had no difficulty with social studies and other subjects for which he was permitted to take his tests orally. Because his writing defied decoding, composition was his weakest subject.

When he reached the 9th grade, Tommy faced new problems. Now, and increasingly since the 6th grade, much of what he was expected to learn required reading and note-taking if he was to meet grade-level expectations. Once again, Tommy was facing frustration and failure. His home-room teacher referred him to the school psychologist for evaluation and possible counseling. Although he was still above average in his intelligence test scores, they showed a 12-point drop[3] and an "uneven" profile.[4] More important than the test scores was the psychologist's observation that she noted numerous expressions of low self-esteem, of statements such as: "This is too hard for me. I'll never be able to do this one." Tommy needed considerable encouragement to "Take a chance and answer as best you can." The psychologist also noted that he was usually correct when he did "take a chance." Tommy also confided that he was having difficulties in getting along with his classmates, much like his problems when he was in the primary grades because he was awkward and could not learn to read and write and his speech was unintelligible. Some of his present classmates called him a "retard" and a few mocked his rapid-fire hard-to-understand speech. Although he admitted that his speech did tend to become unintelligible when he was anxious or in a hurry to get things out, he seldom volunteered to provide answers. However, he had no objection to having his teachers call upon him during class recitations. He still had few friends, and those he had rarely called him by phone. His sister, he noted, spent hours on the telephone. Except for swimming, Tommy admitted that he was definitely a non-athlete.

The plus-side admissions to the psychologist were that he did not doubt that his parents loved him. They tried to assure Tommy that in time he would get over his school difficulties, just as several of his relatives did, including his own father and two uncles and three cousins on his father's side. Even those of his father's relatives who did not progress beyond high school were successful in business. The relatives who did go on to college included two teachers, a physician, a lawyer, and a professor of physics. These relatives, unfortunately for Tommy, all lived in the east, about 3,000 miles from Tommy's home, and so had little contact with him.

Tommy's family decided to transfer him to a private secondary school that specialized in working with students of good intelligence who had learning problems. This school did not have a rigid or "dedicated" approach to remedial reading teaching. Instead, the reading specialist tried out several approaches and adapted one to meet the needs and learning style of each student. In Tommy's instance, the mysteries of the written code were broken and reading became meaningful by an approach that might be characterized as "Look and decide on the likely meaning of the print." In essence, this approach directs that if the reader decides (guesses wrong) because the content fails to make sense and does not relate appropriately to other decoded materials, then he is to reread the lines and find out where he went wrong. If the rereading then makes sense, he goes on. Students are taught the use of the dictionary and are encouraged to check for possible meanings for words that they do not know, or think that they know, but not for the meaning they had in mind. For Tommy, a so-called phonetic (phonemic) approach was ruled out because this had been tried repeatedly and without success throughout his unhappy school career. In addition, Tommy's pronunciations were still too unreliable to permit letter-to-sound (graphemic-phonemic) association.

Tommy blossomed in his new school, both socially and academically. He graduated with a sufficiently high grade-average to be admitted to a California state university, where he majored in mathematics. He went on to earn a Ph.D. in mathematics at a prestigious eastern university. Although Tommy received several offers to teach mathematics at highly rated colleges, he chose instead to accept an appointment to teach in a high school. This decision was motivated by his belief that on a high school level he can be of more help to others like himself who are experiencing failure and frustration as well as social isolation while struggling through school.

Now at age 26, is Tom R. a proficient reader? Judged on accuracy of comprehension, he is; judged on speed of reading, he is not. He does read well enough to manage his local newspaper and most of the *New York Times*. He enjoys reading short stories but admits to having difficulty with the poetry and stories of the *New Yorker*. Except that they tend to be too long, he does better with the feature articles of the *New Yorker*. Tom R. lacks the patience to read full-length novels.[5] Spelling still leaves much to be desired, but his writing is sufficiently legible for him to read what he has written without wondering why he had written it that way in the first place. Fortunately, he seldom has to contend with his penmanship because he has learned to type. His "smart" typewriter that signals him about possible spelling errors is of considerable help.

APPENDIX NOTES

1. Delayed onset of language is a frequent feature of children with developmental dyslexia.

2. Poor motor coordination and late (after age 3) clear expression of hand and general laterality preference associated with persistent unintelligible speech are features of persons who have "cluttered" speech. In some respects the speech component resembles stuttering and is often confused with the latter speech-language problem. Tom's father had also been a clutterer who maintained rapid and often indistinct speech. Cluttering is probably a genetic, male dominant motoric-speech-language complex of improficiencies. Speech production is usually repetitive, fragmented, and too rapid for intelligible articulation. Often reading and writing problems are associated with an early history of cluttering.

3. In conventional intelligence testing, Tom did much better on performance (nonlanguage) items than on those that required language responses. Most

intelligence tests for young children have proportionately more nonverbal (language) items than verbal items. In a later evaluation, Tom's IQ score dropped because of the need to deal with verbal test items.

4. An "uneven" profile is one that shows larger than usual differences between subtest items of a test inventory. A subject with language disabilities or improficiencies is more likely to have an uneven or "scattered" profile than is one without such limitations.

5. Tom's pattern of reading preferences is frequent among adults with a history of dyslexia.

References

Anderson, R. C., & Pearson, P. D. (1985). A schema-theoretic view of basic *processes in reading comprehension*. In P.D. Pearson (Ed.), *Handbook* of reading research (pp. 255–291). New York: Longman.

Anderson, R. C., Hiebert, E. H., Scott, J. A., & Wilkinson, I. A. G (1984). *Becoming a nation of readers: The report of the Commission on Reading.* Washington, DC: National Institute of Education, U. S. Department of Education.

Andrew, J. H. (1981). Reading and cerebral dysfunction among juvenile delinquents. *Criminal Justice and Behavior, 2,* 131–144.

Ashton-Warner, S. (1963). *Teacher.* New York: Simon & Schuster.

Bernstein, B. (1961). Social structure, language, and learning. *Educational Review, 3,* 163–176.

Boder, E. (1973). Developmental dyslexia: A developmental approach based on three atypical reading patterns. *Developmental Medicine and Child Neurology, 15,* 663–687.

Bornstein, H. (1974). Signed English: A manual approach to English language development. *Journal of Speech and Hearing Disorders, 39,* 330–343.

Bornstein, H., & Saulnier, K. L. (1984). *The signed English starter.* Washington, DC: Gallaudet University Press.

Bornstein, H., Saulnier, K. L., & Hamilton, L. B. (Eds.). (1984). *The comprehensive signed English dictionary.* Washington, DC: Gallaudet University Press.

Brown, A. L., Palincsar, A. S., & Armbruster, A. B. (1984). Instructing comprehension-fostering activities in interactive learning situations. In H. Mandl, N. Stein, & T. Trabasso (Eds.), *Learning from texts.* Hillsdale, NJ: Lawrence Erlbaum Associates.

Brown, R. (1973). *A first language: The early stages.* Cambridge: Harvard University Press.

Bruner, J. (1986). *Actual minds, possible worlds.* Cambridge: Harvard University Press.

Calfee, R. C., & Curley, R. G. (1984). Structure of prose in content areas. In J. Flood (Ed.), *Understanding reading comprehension.* Newark, DE: International Reading Association.

Chall, J. S. (1983a). *Learning to read: The great debate.* New York: McGraw-Hill.

Chall, J. S. (1983b). *Stages of reading development.* New York: McGraw-Hill.

Clark, C. R. (1981). Learning words using traditional orthography and the symbols of Rebus, Bliss, and Carrier. *Journal of Speech and Hearing Disorders, 46,* 191–196.

Clark, H., & Clark, E. V. (1977). *Psychology and language.* New York: Harcourt Brace Jovanovich.

Clark, R. (1971). *Einstein, life and times.* New York: World Publishing Company.

Conrad, R. (1977). The reading ability of deaf school leavers. *British Journal of Educational Psychology, 47,* 138–148.

Cox, A. R. (1985). An organization and expansion of Orton-Gillingham. *Annals of Dyslexia, 45,* 187–198.

Critchley, M. (1970). *The dyslexic child.* (2nd ed.). Springfield, IL: Charles C Thomas.

Critchley, M., & Critchley, E. A. (1978). *Dyslexia defined.* London: William Heinemann.

Davis, J. M., & Hardick, E. J. (1981). *Rehabilitative audiology for children and adults.* New York: John Wiley.

Diringer, D. (1968). *The alphabet.* New York: Funk & Wagnalls.

Dolch, E. W. (1960). *Teaching primary reading.* Champaign, IL: Garrard Press.

Downing, J. (1967). *Evaluating the Initial Teaching Alphabet.* London: Cassell.

Eisenson, J. (1984a). *Aphasia and related disorders in children.* New York: Harper & Row.

Eisenson, J. (1984b). *Reading for meaning: An illustrated language acquisition program.* Tulsa, OK: Modern Education Corporation.

Eisenson, J. (1986). *Language and speech disorders in children.* New York: Pergamon Press.

Eisenson, J., & Solomon, H. (1970). Phonemic-graphemic correspondence. Unpublished study.

Fadiman, C. (Ed.). (1985). *The Little, Brown book of anecdotes.* Boston: Little, Brown.

Finucci, J. M., Gottfredson, L. S., & Childs, L. S. (1985). A follow-up study of dyslexic boys. *Annals of Dyslexia, 35,* 117–136.

Gagné, E. D. (1985). *The cognitive psychology of school learning.* Boston: Little, Brown.

Galaburda, A. M. (1985). Developmental dyslexia: A review of biological interactions. *Annals of Dyslexia, 35,* 21–33.

Galbraith, J. K. (1964). *Economic development.* Cambridge: Harvard University Press.

Garner, R., & Reis, R. (1981). Monitoring and resolving comprehension obstacles: An investigation of spontaneous text look-backs among upper grade good and poor comprehenders. *Reading Research Quarterly, 16,* 569–582.

Gates, A. I. (1961). Sex differences in reading ability. *Elementary School Journal, 61,*431–434.

Geschwind, N. (1979). Specializations of the human brain. In *The brain.* San Francisco: W. H. Freeman.

Geschwind, N. (1981). A reaction to the Conference on Sex Differences in Dyslexia. In A. Ansara, N. Geschwind, A. M. Galaburda, M. Albert, & N. Gartrell (Eds.), *Sex differences in dyslexia.* Towson, MD: Orton Dyslexia Society.

Geschwind, N., & Behan, P. (1984). Laterality, hormones, and immunity. In N. Geschwind & A. M. Galaburda (Eds.), *Cerebral dominance: The biological foundations.* Cambridge: Harvard University Press.

Gombrich, E. H (1972). The visual image. *Scientific American, 227,* 82–96.

Gustason, G., Pfetzinger, D., & Azwolkow, E. (1972). *Signing exact English: SEE II.* Rossmoor, CA: Modern Sign Press.

Hansen, J., & Pearson, P.D. (1983). An instructional study: Improving the inferential comprehension of good and poor fourth grade readers. *Journal of Educational Psychology, 75,* 821–829.

Harris, A. J., & Jacobson, M. D. (1975). In A. J. Harris & E. Sipay, *How to increase reading ability.* (5th ed.). New York: David McKay.

Harris, A. J., & Jacobson, M. D. (1972). *Basic elementary reading vocabularies.* New York: Macmillan.

Harris, P. L., Kruithof, M. M., Terwogt, M. M., & Visser, P. (1981). Children's detection and awareness of textual anomaly. *Journal of Experimental Psychology: General, 111,* 414–422.

Hart, B. (1978). Teaching reading to deaf children. New York: Lexington School for the Deaf.

Hehner, B. (1983). *Blissymbolics for use.* Toronto: Blissymbols Communications Institute.

Hier, D. B. (1981). Sex differences in brain structure. In A. Ansara, N. Geschwind, A. M. Galaburda, M. Albert, & N. Gartrell (Eds.), *Sex differences in dyslexia.* Towson, MD: Orton Dyslexic Society.

Hinds, K. (1985). Dyslexia. *Brown University Alumni Magazine,* 25–31.

Hook, P. E., & Johnson, D. D. (1978). Metalinguistic awareness and reading strategies. *Bulletin of the Orton Society, 28,* 63–78.

Johnson, D. D. (1971). The Dolch list re-examined. *The Reading Teacher,* 455–456.

Kamhi, A. G., & Catts, H. W. (1986). Toward an understanding of developmental language and reading disorders. *Journal of Speech and Hearing Disorders, 51,* 337–347.

Kretschmer, R., & Kretschmer, L. (1978). *Language development and intervention with the hearing impaired.* Baltimore: University Park Press.

LaBerge, D., & Samuels, S. J. (1974). Toward a theory of automatic information processing in reading. *Cognitive psychology, 6,* 293–323.

Loring, J. M. & Loring, L. (1982). *Pictographs and petroglyphs.* Los Angeles: University of California Institute of Archeology.

Maccoby, E. (1966). *Development of sex differences.* Stanford, CA: Stanford University Press.

Maccoby, E., & Jacklin, C. (1974). *Psychology of sex differences.* Stanford, CA: Stanford University Press.

Masland, R. L. (1981). Summary of the conference proceedings. In A. Ansara, N. Geschwind, A. M. Galaburda, M. Albert, & N. Gartrell (Eds.), *Sex differences in dyslexia.* Towson, MD: Orton Dyslexia Society.

Mattis, S., French, J. H. & Rapin, I. (1975). Dyslexia in children and young adults. *Developmental Medicine and Child Neurology, 17,* 150–161.

Mayer, R. E. (1980). Elaboration techniques that increase the meaningfulness of technical text: An experimental test of the learning strategy hypothesis. *Journal of Educational Psychology, 72,* 770–784.

Mayer, R. E. (1983). Can you repeat that? Qualitative effects of repetition and advance organizers on learning science prose. *Journal of Educational Psychology, 75,* 40–49.

Mazurkiewicz, A. J. (1966). *The Initial Teaching Alphabet and the world of English.* In L. Dunn, M. S. Mueller, & M. D. Neely, *The efficacy of the Initial Teaching Alphabet and the Peabody Language Development Kit with grade one disadvantaged children.* Hempstead, NY: Hofstra University, Initial Teaching Alphabet Foundation.

Mazurkiewicz, A. J. (1973). The I.T.A. revisited. Paper presented at annual meeting of the College Reading Association, November.

Menyuk, P., & Flood, J. (1981). Language development, reading/writing problems and remediation. *Bulletin of the Orton Society, 31,* 13–28.

Meyer, B. J. F. (1975). *The organization of prose and its effects on memory.* Amsterdam: North-Holland Publishing Co.

Meyer, B. J. F. (1977). The structure of prose: Effects on learning and memory and implications for educational practice. In R. C. Anderson, R. J. Spiro, & W. J. Montague (Eds.), *Schooling and the acquisition of knowledge.* Hillsdale, NJ: Lawrence Erlbaum Associates.

*Meyer, B. J. F. (1985). Prose analysis: Purposes, procedures, and problems. In B. K. Britton & J. B. Black (Eds.), *Understanding expository text.* Hillsdale, NJ: Lawrence Erlbaum Associates.

*Meyer, B. J. F., Brandt, B. F., & Bluth, G. J. (1980). Use of top-level structure in text: Key for reading comprehension of ninth-grade students. *Reading Research Quarterly, 16,* 72–103.

*Meyer, T. J. (1986). America's costliest college. *Chronicle of Higher Education, 31,* 30–31.

Mittenthal, S. (1986). Kindergarten: Starting older and wiser. *New York Times,* November 20, 1986.

Morgan, J. (1984). *Agatha Christie: A biography.* London: Collins.

Mulligan, W. (1969). A study of dyslexia and delinquency. *Academic Therapy, 4,* 177–187.

Norton, W. T. (1975). Myelin. In D. B. Tower, *The nervous system.* Vol. 1. New York: Raven Press.

Ornstein, R., & Thompson, R. F. (1984). *The amazing brain.* Boston: Houghton Mifflin.

Pearson, P. D., & Johnson, D. D. (1977). *Teaching reading comprehension.* New York: Holt, Rinehart & Winston.

Pirozzolo, F. J. (1979). *The neuropsychology of developmental reading disorders.* New York: Praeger.

Potter, B. (1904). *The tale of Benjamin Bunny* (pp. 22–29). New York: Frederick Warne and Co.

Professional Seminar Consultants. (1978). *P.S.C. Information Manual.* Oceanside, NY. Author.

Quigley, S., & King. C. (1984). *Reading milestones.* Beaverton, OR: Dormac.

Quigley, S., & Paul, P. V. (1984). *Language and deafness.* San Diego, CA: College Hill Press.

Rayner, K. (1983). Eye movement, perceptual span, and reading disability. *Annals of Dyslexia, 33,* 163–173.

Roswell, F. G., & Natchez, G. (1977). *Reading disability.* (3rd ed.). New York: Basic Books.

Rozin, P., Poritsky, S., & Sotsky, R. (1971). American children with reading problems can easily learn to read English represented by Chinese characters. *Science, 171,* 1264–1267.

Ryan, E. B., & Ledger, G. W. (1978). *Differences in syntactic skills between good and poor readers in the first grade.* (ERIC Microfiche No. ED176232).

Sartre, P. (1981). *The family idiot (a biography of Gustave Flaubert).* Chicago: University of Chicago Press.

Simpson, E. (1979). *Reversals: A personal account of victory over dyslexia.* Boston: Houghton Mifflin.

Smith, E. B., Goodman, K. S., & Meredith, R. (1976). *Language and thinking in school.* (2nd ed). New York: Holt, Rinehart & Winston.

Spache, G. D. (1976). *Investigating the issues of reading disabilities.* Boston: Allyn & Bacon.

Springer, S. P., & Deutsch, G. (1981). *Left brain, right brain.* New York: W. H. Freeman.

Stanovich, K. E. (1985). Explaining the variance of reading ability in terms of psychological processes. *Annals of Dyslexia,* 67–96.

Stein, N. L., & Glenn, C. G. (1979). An analysis of story comprehension in elementary school children. In L. Freedle (Ed.), *New directions in discourse processing.* Norwood, NJ: Ablex.

Stewart, R. W., & Huber, J. (1966). Two years with I.T.A. In A. J. Mazurkiewicz, *The Initial Teaching Alphabet and the world of English.* Hempstead, NY: Hofstra University, Initial Teaching Alphabet Foundation.

Thomas, L. (1975). *The lives of a cell* (pp. 111–112). New York: Bantam Books.

Thompson, L. L. (1979). Language disabilities in men of eminence. *Journal of Learning Disabilities, 4,* 39–50.

Thomson, M. E. (1984). *Developmental dyslexia.* London: Edward Arnold.

Tierney, R. J., & Cunningham, J. W. (1984). Research on teaching reading comprehension. In P. D. Pearson (Ed.), *Handbook of reading research* (pp. 609–655). New York: Longman.

Vellutino, F. R. (1979). *Dyslexia: Theory and research.* Cambridge: MIT Press.

Vellutino, F. R. (1983). Childhood dyslexia: A language disorder. In H. Myklebust (Ed.), *Progress in learning disabilities.* New York: Grune and Stratton.

Weinstein, C. E., Underwood, V. L., Wicker, F. W., & Cubberly, W. E. (1979). Cognitive learning strategies: Verbal and imaginal elaboration. In H. F. O'Neill, Jr. & D. C. Spielberger (Eds.), *Cognitive and affective learning strategies.* New York: Academic Press.

Williams, J. (1979). Reading instruction today. *American Psychologist, 3,* 917–922.

Woodcock, R. W., & Clark, C. R. (1969). *Peabody Rebus Reading Program.* Circle Pines, MN: American Guidance Service.

Yeats, W. B. (1926). *Autobiographies.* London: Macmillan.

Young, P., & Tyre, C. (1983). *Dyslexia or illiteracy?* Stony Stratford, England: The Open University Press.

Index